God's Miracle

A Story of Faith in the Face of Loss

by Darlene Wiebe

ISBN

978-1-4602-4468-5 (Hardcover)

978-1-4602-4469-2 (Paperback)

978-1-4602-4470-8 (eBook)

Produced by:

FriesenPress

Suite 300 — 852 Fort Street

Victoria, BC, Canada V8W 1H8

www.friesenpress.com

Distributed to the trade by The Ingram Book Company

Foreword

It is my hope this book will bring hope and comfort to parents who have lost a child, regardless of age, be it pre-natal or post-natal. Others want to comfort and do their best but they sometimes don't understand the depth of grief that comes from a loss in very early pregnancy and/or how to respond to it. Finding professional and/or group support is important to coming to terms with the loss and the need to grieve. It has helped me gain a perspective that has helped me move forward in peace and faith.

—Darlene Wiebe, March 2014

Dedication

Tirzah — the reason that I get up most mornings. You are the light of my life and mean the world to me. I pray that you will never forget how special you are because God rewrote the medical books when you were born, my medical miracle. I love you!!

Rob — the love of my life. We have been through the process of grieving and coping together and at the same time have journeyed on very different paths. You meant it when you said "in sickness or health till death do us part." You have been there on the days when I was a hormonal basket case and not able to make decisions, or have been double guessing decisions made. You lost your children too and I want to acknowledge your losses. I know you are hurting too. We have grown closer, not further apart, through all that we have experience together and for that I am extremely grateful.

To my eight children that I will always hold in my heart even though I have never held you in my arms - Kipp, Adriel, Litonya, Jezaniah, Nika, Shala, Rena & Mara. I'm looking forward to seeing you in heaven.

Chapter 1

My parents were married on May 4th, 1968. A little less than a year later on March 25th, 1969 my brother, Daniel Dale, was stillborn at seven months gestation. Mommy had started bleeding or so they thought. They realized too late it was actually Daniel who was bleeding. By the time they discovered this he had bled to death. Looking back, we think Mommy may have had Type O negative blood because she had no trouble with her other two pregnancies. As adults, we discovered both Debbie and I have Type O negative blood and we know Dad has O positive. This may well have been the cause of Daniel's death, although it is unusual for this to happen with the first pregnancy.

I was born on June 2nd, 1970 at the Johnson Memorial Hospital in Gimli, Manitoba at about 12:30 p.m. My full given name is Esther Darlene. Both names were very intentional.

Esther was the name of my Mommy's youngest sister. She had been a baby when their mother passed away. My grandfather could not look after all nine children by himself, so the youngest five were 'farmed out' to other families that were able to care for them. When my grandfather remarried, all but the youngest child came back to live with him and his new wife. The youngest was adopted by the family she had been staying with for reasons I was never told. I am not sure if the stepmother did not want this child or if they felt the child had been so young at the time she went to live with the family that it would be cruel to take her away because that was the only family she had really ever known.

Whatever the reason, Mommy always was very resentful of that decision. In her grown years, Mommy maintained very close contact with this sister, who died before I was born. I was named after her.

My dad tells me they chose Darlene because it was the closest to darling they could get in a name. I am glad they had the sense to not make my middle name Darling! I was 3.222 kg (7 lbs 2 oz) at birth and 53.5 cm (21") long. You could not have pinched my cheeks as I was a baby with no extra fat on me. I was born into a practicing Christian family. God was and is still very important to them.

My Grandma Friesen has faithfully prayed for her family every day for many years. The answers to her prayers are evident in the fact that almost all of her fourteen children are serving the Lord either in full time ministry or in reaching out to people in their work places.

Among the grandchildren and great grandchildren all but a handful are living for the Lord and many are involved in missions as well. Grandma may have lived on a farm in the middle of nowhere raising children but the ripple effect of her enduring faith has been seen and felt around the world. Some of the countries she has touched are Canada, United States, Mexico, Cuba, Jamaica, Dominican Republic, Guatemala, Belize, Nicaragua, Bolivia, Chili, Paraguay, Ireland, England, United Kingdom, Norway, Sweden, Poland, Netherlands, Germany, Ukraine, Moldova, Romania, Yugoslavia, Kosovo, Bulgaria, Albania, Greece, Portugal, Malta, Tunisia, Egypt, Israel, Ethiopia, Congo, Kenya, Uganda, Zimbabwe, Mozambique, South Africa, Georgia, Russia, Tajikistan,

Pakistan, India, Nepal, Thailand, Singapore, Central Asia, Australia and Philippines. This list may not be complete, and will probably be expanded in the future; but as of right now there has been someone from Grandma's family on every continent except Greenland. And these are just the ones to which her direct descendants went. In many cases, they touched people's lives there who came from many other countries. Never underestimate the power of prayer. And thank God for fourteen children because my grandparents could reach many more places than if they had chosen to have a smaller family.

We lived right next to Grandma and Grandpa Friesen, about eleven kilometers (seven miles) north of Riverton Manitoba in a community called Mennville. My dad's youngest brother Roy was just a year and a half older than I was and we were very close from as early as I can remember. We spent many hours playing together as the two properties were separated by only a hedge. We were either outside or at each other's houses most of the time. Being in the country, our next nearest neighbours lived half a mile away but they did not have any children our age. So, as children Roy and I were each other's playmates and as teens he was my big brother who protected and looked out for me. No boy dared mess with me because of him.

One situation I remember well was when I was attending the public school in town for grades eleven and twelve. Some of the guys in school were harassing me about something , in a way that I was pretty sure was very crude. I asked Roy what they were referring to. Roy was almost embarrassed to tell me but he did because he knew I needed to know, so I could have one up on them. When I went to school the next day and they approached me, I was ready. I told them in no uncertain terms they were to leave me alone and gave them the definition of the term they were using. They were shocked and royally embarrassed to have a Mennonite girl explaining a sexual act to them. They wanted to know who had told me and I told them it was my Uncle Roy who had graduated from Riverton the year before. I was never again harassed in the same way and it seemed like there was a level of respect for me among the masses from that day on.

Roy was my escort for my grad two years later, much to the dismay of many of my female classmates as many of them had no escort (and the fact that many of them had had a crush on him when he was in Riverton didn't help). To this day we have a connection that is closer to brother and sister than uncle and niece. It was a sad day in my life when he and his family moved overseas. I have missed them a lot.

I do not have many memories of Grandpa Friesen but the ones I do have are very vivid and have been confirmed by others as actually taking place. I remember going over to see him often. With only a hedge separating our houses it was easy to do even as a toddler. On those occasions I played with Uncle Roy. Grandpa was already not well by this time and I would often just sit in his room by his bed on a little home-made wooden stool. I don't recall that much was ever said. One other thing I remembered about their house at the time was that they had installed a flush toilet. I found out later that this was because Grandpa could not deal with the smell of the cash and carry variety. This was way before its time in our community.

When he was taken to the hospital for the last time before he died, I remember Roy and I sat with him on the floor of their vehicle while he lay in the back seat. The last time I saw him was through the hospital window. I remember how much I missed him. I was visiting at my uncle and aunt's in Gimli. My aunt held me up to the window (he was on ground level) so that I could see him again. I was too young to go into his room (how things have changed). He saw me from the far bed and with a smile blew me a kiss. That was the last time I saw him alive. To my recollection he passed away within a month after that on September 8th, 1972.

On January 22nd, 1973 I lost my single child status. I was not old enough to remember when Debbie was born or the events around her birth, although I have been told I really did not want to give up my position as the baby. In my mind she has always been there, even though the calendar tells us she is two and a half years younger than me. As we grew, this did not changed and today we are very close and it seems that we can almost read each other's minds sometimes. Throughout the next few years I had what I considered a normal childhood. Nothing significant happened.

My Grandpa Dueck was killed in a car accident on June 20th, 1976. When I heard the news that where Grandpa had been killed, Mommy, Debbie and I were in the graveyard where Grandma Dueck was buried. We were doing some weeding on the graves belonging to Mommy's family. I do not know who found us there and told us. I just remember our next stop was the location of the car.

The windshield was busted badly. It seemed surreal. But I now had only one grandma left. I had just turned six. Looking back I realize how important grandparents are in a child's life and wish I had not lost three of mine so young. As with my Grandpa Friesen, I was close to my Grandpa Dueck. I remember many times he came to visit. We even had a roughed out room where he stayed when he came. Those were exciting times for Debbie and myself. When he died there was a hole in my life. I so missed my grandpas.

My Uncle Dave (Mommy's brother) filled the role at this point and became my Grandpa. We went to visit Uncle Dave and Aunt Katherine often. Uncle Dave was fun-loving and I probably loved the visits at their house more than any others. He always had time for us and seemed to have energy to match ours. Looking back, I realize he actually sat most of the time but the games he could play while doing that were amazing.

Aunt Katherine was an amazing cook, or at least I thought so. My favourite was when we would visit in summer and have watermelon and *Roul Kooke* (the Low German word for a deep fried non-sweet fritter) to our heart's content. Forget supper ! ... or was that supper?

When I was eight years old Uncle Dave had a very bad accident. He pulled through against all odds, but was permanently disabled. Despite this, anytime he was told he couldn't, he set out to prove he could.

When he was told that Parkinson's Disease would probably set in within a few years, he asked the doctor what he could do and was told keeping active would delay the onset. He walked almost daily and created projects he could work on till they moved into the 55Plus unit. It took the Parkinson's more than thirty years to set in, and even when it did he determinedly still walked for about four miles, at least three to five times a week.

Until the day he went into a semi-comatose state the nursing staff had to forever keep their eyes on him because he would still try to do things he could in reality no longer do.

Chapter 2

On the morning of April 22nd, 1981 I was feeling sick again. This was not unusual as I was sick a lot in my early years. By lunch I was feeling better, so off to school I went. I had missed a lot of school already that year and Mommy felt I needed to go to school for the afternoon. Many times throughout the years I wish I had not felt better. As she dropped me off I kissed her good-bye and walked into the school. That was the last time I saw her alive. She stopped in on the way home to pick up a carding machine from a lady in the community. As she came to the Number Eight Highway crossing a mile and a half from home, she failed to stop at a stop sign and was T-boned on the passenger side at one hundred kilometers (sixty-three mles) per hour by a truck.

The road would have been very familiar to her and we think she must not have been paying attention, because she realized where she was a few seconds before the stop sign. We know this because there were tire skid marks from a few feet before the stop sign onto the pavement to where the car came to a rest on the shoulder. The truck that T-boned the car slid into the ditch.

She was killed instantly. Delbert Brandt (a young man who lived near the scene of the accident) had been delayed and was just leaving for work when the accident occurred. He recognized the car immediately, went back home and told his mom to call Dad. He returned to the scene of the accident. Dad arrived on the scene within fifteen minutes of the collision and was met there by Delbert. The car was banged up so badly that the passenger side was pushed in to where the driver's side should have been. When Dad walked over to the car, he saw Mommy lying on the shoulder, having fallen out of the seat when the car stopped. He looked for me in the back seat and when he saw the carding machine he knew I was at school and not at the crash site. Mommy had blood coming out of her mouth, so he knew she was gone. He then walked over to the truck to see if they were all right.

Someone had already brought some blankets for them. He gave them a Gideon New Testament and left. It was only after he left that they were told he was the husband of the woman that they had just hit. There were three people in the truck; two of them were getting married the following weekend. They were all taken to hospital, examined and released with the greatest injury being a broken leg. To our knowledge the engaged couple became believers because of what Dad did.

Emergency vehicles had been called and they arrived a short time later. It took over two hours for the mess to be cleaned up. Leonard Dueck (Mommy's cousin's husband, they lived in the community) drove Dad to school to pick us up at about 2:15 p.m. There were already quite a number of people gathered at Grandma's by that time, as news in a small rural community travels fast. It was just the beginning of recess when Lorna, Roy, Debbie and I were picked up. The teachers had already been notified about the accident. I am not sure how they managed to come back to class and be normal. We were all puzzled at this turn of events.

When Dad told us our Mommy was in heaven, I remember thinking he must mean Grandma. He told us there had been an accident and it appeared she had died instantly. They took the long way home because they were not sure if the accident had been cleaned up yet. We did not return to school till after the funeral. Later that evening we went to the scene of the accident in our truck, now the only vehicle we had. We saw the skid marks our car had made and saw the exact point of contact as they made a ninety degree turn on the highway and started moving along the highway instead of across it. We knew where it had come to rest because we could see the big puddle of blood where Mommy had fallen out of the vehicle.

The other tracks went into the ditch and the grass was all packed down where the pick-up truck had stopped. That night, Grandma's house was full to the brim with relatives. All the younger unmarried aunts and the girl cousins slept in the rec-room downstairs at Grandma's. We joined them. Dad went home and I am sure our bed was occupied by another relative. I remember laying down close to Aunt Lorna (Dad's youngest sister) that night and it hitting me that I no longer had a mother.

The tears came and flowed for a long time till sleep took over. The next couple of days were a blur. I know many tears were shed. I do not remember going to our house before the funeral but I'm sure I did. However, I slept at my Grandma's house until the day of the funeral. Sharon Friesen, a lady from our church, came by Grandma's twice with enough baking to feed a large crowd. She said she was sure there were many people coming and going and she wanted to help Grandma to be certain that anyone that dropped by could have a snack.

Dad took Debbie and me with him when it was time to make the funeral arrangements. We went with Klassens Funeral Home and this started a long-term relationship with the owner/operator. Dad said Debbie and I could pick out the casket. The one we picked was probably the cheapest one on the floor. It was a pink cloth one. The viewing took place on April 26th in the evening at the funeral home in the city of Winnipeg (the nearest city to our area). Walking in, I remember being upset about how Mommy looked. They had not done her hair like she usually had it and she did not look like herself. I walked out and I am not sure how they changed it to her usual style so quickly but sometime between the family viewing and the public viewing the hair was changed and I settled down.

The funeral was on April 27th. I don't remember much of it, but I know I shed no tears that day. I thought something was wrong and my Aunt Lorna told me it was okay. She said I just had no more tears to cry right now. I slept through the service and to this day have never heard the service in its entirety. I had always meant to listen to the tape of it but never had time. Now I have no desire to do so.

It was probably the biggest funeral up to that time in the Mennville Evangelical Mennonite Church. I remember walking out after the funeral to the graveside. The auditorium, foyer and basement were full of people and there were quite a few standing outside on the front cement pad and listening from there.

Life changed drastically as we started trying to figure out our new normal. Sadly, this event changed our relationship with Grandma. She stepped in and started to act like a mother and this did not work out too well, even though she meant well. This was a role though that she continued to try and push herself into even after Mom (my dear stepmother) and Dad got married.

It was frustrating for us and I am sure Mom was probably frustrated as well. During the time between Mommy's death and Dad remarrying we ate the majority of our suppers at Grandma's. I guess this was a good thing because I am not sure how well we would have eaten if it were up to Dad or myself. We might have lived on porridge, peanut butter and cheese sandwiches, and fried eggs. I am grateful to my Grandma Friesen for the care she did give us. I just sometimes wish she had stuck to meeting our physical needs and left the parenting to Dad. It was hard enough losing a mother, but to essentially 'lose' my only remaining grandparent was also hard. Sadly, it seemed that this was a role that she could never quite give up.

During this time when Debbie and I were motherless, we became even closer. I took on the role of mother to a point. I felt the need to look out for her and protect her somehow.

Chapter 3

In June, Dad told us he was going to ask a young woman out. When he said who she was, we didn't have a clue who he was talking about until he mentioned she was the blonde-haired lady we occasionally gave a ride to from church to her parents' place. Our response was "Oh, that pretty lady." I do not exactly remember if he asked if we were okay with it or not. I think it was just a fact.

'Mom' had grown up in the community but was now in Three Hills, Alberta at Prairie Bible College as a dean of women. Dad had written her a letter in May but a mail strike had prevented him from receiving her response to his thirteen-page letter. Her twin brother was getting married in July and she had planned to come out for that but because of Dad's letter she almost cancelled her plans. We met her sometime in July of that year. She and Dad had already been on a date, which we had heard him arrange from Grandma's rec-room. It went fairly well I think. I do not remember much about the visit.

She headed back to the Bible college in about the middle of August. As I and my sister got to know her over the next couple of months we started getting excited about the possibility of another mother. We never talked on the phone but letters were exchanged. Sometimes Dad would even read us sections of his to us. The truth be told, we were sick of Grandma acting like we needed a parent. We still had Dad but Grandma stepped in far too often to establish the law. On more than one occasion Dad had to tell her he was still the parent and she did not have that authority.

'Mom' came home again at Christmas. On the evening of December 22nd, I had a sleepover at my friend's house because Dad was out on a date. The next evening when we got home from school Dad told us he had proposed and that 'Mom' had accepted. Later that evening she came over and after some discussion it was decided she would go by Mom to differentiate between our biological mother and her. To this day she is Mom and if we talk about Mommy we all know we are talking about our biological mother.

We were told we should not tell anyone about the engagement for a couple of days. I am not sure of the reasoning behind it, but it was a big order for two young girls who were excited about it especially because school was still in session. The evening after the engagement was the annual school Christmas program. Mom and Dad sat near the back of the church together and I think this was the first indication to most of the church that there was a relationship between the two of them. After Christmas Mom went back to Three Hills to finish out the year.

Over the next six months we got ready for the change. During this time Grandma tried to be helpful and told us all sorts of things Mom would expect and what she was like. We didn't put much stock in her words and it was a good thing. Grandma was wrong on most counts. One of the things Grandma was most adamant about was that Mom would never allow cats in the house or in the playhouse. I am sure she told us this because she did not like animals in the house and she thought this would stop us from bringing them in.

I am not sure how Grandma made out with Mommy or maybe she didn't know because Mommy loved animals in the house and on many occasions we would have eight or more cats in the house at one time. When Mom arrived at our house in mid June, she arrived with a house cat. Grandma was silenced.

Mom and Dad were married on June 26th, 1982 and we were the honourary candle lighters because the Reimer grandparents didn't approve of candles. The exchange of rings was also too worldly and Mom and Dad did not exchange rings until afterwards when they were not present. For years, they would remove their rings in the car before going into Grandma and Grandpa's Reimer's house.

The wedding included an acceptance ceremony of Mom acknowledging us as daughters. The full acceptance however did not take place till the fall of 1985 after she came back from a conference. She had come home late the night before and we were already in bed. The next day we got up to go to school and we were told we would be going later. As our family sat at the kitchen table (a great bonding place) Mom told us she was home. We asked for clarification because it seemed like the obvious fact because she was sitting there with us. She explained that at the conference her heart had been changed. Inwardly she had still been thinking about the mission field that she had never arrived at. Now she knew and was choosing to be content on the farm. She had 'unpacked' and she was home. The change was very obvious to us, but only last year was I made aware by Roy that the change had also been noticed by the relatives still living at home with Grandma Friesen. They had always wondered what had happened.

The collision of cultures had started. Debbie and I were pre-teen now and the difference between the Friesen family and the Reimer family could not have been more different. It was an adjustment that took years to make, and sometimes I am not sure if I have yet entirely made it. To this day I feel most of the family accepts us but it is more of a friendship as adult peers than real family. Maybe this is only my perception because of the way we were treated by Grandma Reimer and she may just have been a poor filter. Maybe it is because of our age when Mom and Dad got married. And maybe the family cultures we had had up to that point were so different that we just could not fit the groove this family was trying to put us in.

There are two of Mom's siblings that are married to my cousins and our relationship stayed more like cousins than uncle/aunt and niece. Debbie and I were continually in the hot seat for what we did (hair length, using make-up and jewellery, using the wrong colors, etc.). We were told in many ways that we were a very bad influence within the family — we were told directly, and also in the context of children's stories at Christmas that were directed more at us than at the children. This got hard and the walls were built.

Mom expected us to wear certain things to her parents' place, which we resisted a lot. This often forced Dad to play the mediator between us and Mom. As I got older I realized that what was actually happening was that it was a demonstration of respect to Grandma and Grandpa to wear dresses. I look back and realize Mom was probably getting a lot of flak from her mom about us and our worldliness. I'm sorry Mom for all the grief that I caused you during this time. I just didn't understand. When I realized years later that Grandma talked to Mom about my choices I told Mom she needed to tell Grandma to talk to me because I was now an adult and responsible for my own choices.

We were directly accused of leading the other younger cousins astray, including when two of them had children out of wedlock. I am still not sure how we accomplished this by cutting our hair and using make-up. As I got older I tried to show respect to my grandparents but I also respectfully chose to be true to me when I kept my purity ring on and had my hair shorter than they would have liked. I explained to Grandma one day after she critically pointed out the ring again, that I wore the ring as a promise to myself to save sex till marriage. That was the last time that she said anything about it.

Later she told me that afterward, when she saw the ring on my hand, she was glad I was standing strong on Godly morals. Too bad for all those years she spent nagging at the outward things her family was doing wrong. If only she had chosen to focus and speak to her family about the things that really mattered.

At Grandpa's funeral in July 2011 as family shared their experiences and memories of Grandpa I was saddened and cried a little. I realized I had not known him at all. I knew Grandma and realized then that Grandma had been the driving force in the negative environment we were introduced into. Grandpa had sat on the sidelines and let Grandma rule. How I wish Grandpa had gotten off the sidelines and been the Grandpa I so badly needed him to be. I am sure my experiences in the family would have been very different if Grandpa spoken for himself instead of letting Grandma do it — sometimes through him.

It seemed when the others shared their stories it was almost always times when they had been with Grandpa alone, an opportunity I never had.

The one memory that sticks out in my mind about Grandpa is one Sunday afternoon when the larger family was sitting around the kitchen table eating Faspa. I told this joke. If a train crashed on the Canada/US border, where would the survivors be buried? The discussion that followed was intense as everyone tried to figure it out. Grandpa on the other hand was sitting at the end of the table smirking as he made eye contact with me. He had it figured out right away.

There was one thing I always did looked forward to when we went to visit the Reimer Grandparents. Grandma Reimer was an awesome cook. I would choose her food over Grandma Friesen's any day.

When Mom and Dad told us Mom was pregnant, we were excited. Once again we were told not to tell anyone. Apparently we were a very secretive family. Not much was discussed beyond that for the remainder of the pregnancy. I hoped Mom would let me feel the baby move but that didn't happen. The other thing that didn't happen was being told the due date. I found out when I heard Mom tell an aunt on the Reimer side. This hurt because I felt that, if it was in fact information that could be shared with a few select people, why were we not in this group?

Mom went into labour on a Saturday night. The next morning Debbie and I were awakened by an aunt and told that Mom and Dad had gone to the hospital. We went to church that morning and then to Grandma Friesen's for the afternoon. We got the call sometime between three and four in the afternoon of May 22nd, 1983 that Rebekah had arrived safe and sound.

There was one damper to all this. We found out Grandma Friesen had been calling the hospital about every half hour to see how things were going. She had been told by the nurses before Dad called us that a baby girl had been born. This angered Debbie and me. We expressed this to Dad and he said it would be different next time.

We went to see Rebekah for the first time on Monday. The room for women who'd had their babies was at the end of a long hallway from the hospital entrance. We were waiting in the entrance and saw Mom at the door holding Rebekah. We knew the hospital was not a place to run, but run we did. The hallway made a perfect indoor track.

I was baptized by pouring on June 9th, 1985. This is a good thing because of an earlier experience with water. To this day, I have a good chance of losing it entirely if someone else gets my face wet. If immersion had been the only option, I am pretty sure I would still not have taken the step of water baptism. I do not recall having any wild emotions during or after the event. I just knew that as a believer the Bible commanded it.

When Mom and Dad told us she was pregnant again, we were not surprised. We had been old enough when Rebekah was born to figure out the signs of pregnancy. Again, they would not tell us when the baby was due. After some quick calculations we figured it out and approached them about it. We were bang on with the due date. They were very surprised and asked us how we had figured it out. As the pregnancy progressed we asked them if it was twins. They told us "God hadn't told them yet." We didn't buy the answer and assumed twins.

This time, true to their word, Grandma did not find out Mom had gone to the hospital. Rebekah had been picked up by Aunt Kathy (Mom's sister-in-law) and when we got home from school on March 20th, 1986 we knew instantly where Mom and Dad were. Lunch was on the table but hardly touched. We got a call from Aunt Kathy saying that Rebekah was at their house, because Mom and Dad had had to go to Gimli. We thanked her for the information.

That evening we got call after call from Grandma asking for Dad. She wanted to know if Roy was needed on the farm that evening. We told her Mom and Dad had gone to Gimli to finalize the car deal from earlier in the week and we were sure that Dad didn't have anything urgent that needed doing or else he would have left a list. Later, Roy came by because Grandma had told him to check just to make sure. We told him where they actually were but told him not to tell Grandma. He didn't.

That evening we could not sleep. We must have dozed in the living room because we woke up very quickly when Dad came in at 3 a.m. He had not called from the hospital because we had a party line back then and Grandma had a habit of picking up the phone and listening in. He told us we had another sister and at the same time Debbie and I asked "and?" He was surprised we seemed to know as he claimed he and Mom had not even known till a month previous. "And a brother," was his response.

After that we tried to get some sleep before school the next day. In the morning before we went to school he called Grandma and we listened in. Grandma was so upset because one — something could have happened to Mom (like she was able to do anything about it if it had) and two — we had lied to her (which was partly true but all we had been told by Aunt Kathy is that they had gone to Gimli and the car was the alibi we used so she wouldn't be minding our business). We went to see Mom that evening and were introduced to Judith and Jason.

Chapter 4

The big day came. I had attended a small private school for the first ten years and for the last two I had transferred to the public school in Riverton. School was never easy for me. I struggled to pass every subject and even then there were a few I failed. If I came home with even a 'D', I was thankful. I was never an 'A' student. I managed to pass each grade but I am not entirely sure the teachers didn't sometimes arrange that.

I started Grade one speaking only Low German and had a less than working knowledge of English. This presented some challenges because there was a rule in school that the students could not speak Low German as some of the teachers didn't know it. If you did speak it you got your name on the board and demerits started being added for every new infraction. I shut up and still got my name on the board because I was now not co-operating. A visit from my parents quickly solved the problem and I was given an exception to the rule as I learned the English language. I am not sure this made me very popular with the other students but I think most of them understood.

I did not have very many friends during my school years and was alone much of the time. I was often teased and even at times physically bullied. The reasons I was teased were many — I had old parents, I was forced to eat vitamins at home, my hair and clothes were outdated, my lunches were gross, I had small feet, I sucked at sports, my first name was fun to mock, etc.

I learned early to fight back. Eventually, I had the respect of most of the other students but did not have friends. By nature I was shy and timid and a very petite girl but I learned early that to survive, I would need to earn respect.

There are a few very clear memories I have about school. The first one happened in Grade one. Our grade had been sent downstairs to work with flashcards. Kenton and I were in a group. We were diligently doing our work when Kenton had a really stinky fart. We moved location and the other group tattled on us. Later, I realized it was probably because they had been goofing off and were scared we would report them because an aunt who had been in the class above where the other two girls were 'working' said they had been really loud and their teacher had had to go downstairs and tell them to be quiet.

We were hauled upstairs and told that for not doing our work we were going to get a spanking. I had never been so mortified in my life. I was in tears before I was even hit with the ruler over the hand in front of the entire class. There was no chance given for an explanation. The teacher never apologized to us although I am sure he was corrected. He lost any respect he might have had from the students that day, not only in our classroom but in the rest of the school as well. He did not return to teach the next year.

Another thing I clearly remember happened in Grade four. As usual, I was really struggling in math and finally gave up and took answers from another student. The teacher caught me and became upset with me. When I burst into tears she softened and took me into the staff room. Unlike the time in Grade one with the other teacher, she took the time to see if there was an underlying problem. When I told her I just didn't understand how to do it, she made sure I had some extra help.

In the small private school there were three to four grades in a class taught by one teacher. They did the best they could but educational assistants did not exist there. Grade five was a rough year because that was the year Mommy was killed in the car accident and I missed a couple of weeks of school. For someone who already struggles in anything academic this did not make for an easy year, as I missed so much class instruction time. Thankfully, my aunt took on the task of being a tutor and I probably did the best I ever had in any other grade. This aunt went on to get her teaching degree and became an awesome teacher based on Debbie's reports (she had her as a teacher in high school for a few years).

My teacher also was a Godsend that year. She was hands down the best teacher I had in my first ten grades. She had the full respect of the students in the entire school. During my absence those couple of weeks, she streamlined my homework requirements so I got the gist of what I missed.

In Grade seven, I had a day when I was feeling sick but was in school anyway. A guy from two grades above me came over and put his arm around me. I lost it. I was holding a pencil at the time and with that pencil attacked him. I had him bending backwards over a desk and was stabbing at him with the pencil. My uncle, who was also in the class, pulled me off. Later I heard I had gotten pretty close to his eye with one of my stabs.

We were having revival meetings at our church that week and at the service that night Dad happened to hear (from the boy's father I believe) what had happened at school that day. Dad came home and asked if the report was true. When I said it was, he was shocked that I would have actually fought with someone, never mind a guy older than me.

That night was a turning point in my life. I had prayed the prayer of salvation at about age four. That night I asked God to be my Saviour and Lord again, based on a more complete knowledge of what I was committing to. The next day my fellow classmate apologized for being mean the previous day and I forgave him. Another time in this same grade there was a group of us out in the bush that was on the located at the edge of the school yard. It was a place where many a lunch hour was spent by the students. Someone had found a pack of smokes and decided they were going to try their hand at smoking. I had the misfortune of being with the group that day. I didn't want to but they pressured me to try and because I already felt like I was not accepted in the group I caved.

The next day my Uncle Roy told me that the teachers found out about it through one of the parents. I guess one of the students had told their parents about it. I was not in school that day (probably sick) and missed the individual interrogation every student received. My dad found out about it and was so proud of me that I had not done it. Apparently, none of the students had given my name as one that was involved or it was assumed that I was a good little girl who never got in trouble. I told him that was not true; I had in fact been with the group and had tried. But I assured him and Mom I would never touch another cigarette as long as I lived. It had been gross and disgusting and I had more brains than to force myself to try to like it.

This grade must have been a difficult one because there is one more memory I have about it. We needed to write a paper on the novel *Jean val Jean*. I had been carefully taking notes and a few days before the paper was due, my rough copy was stolen. I frantically rewrote the paper and managed to finish it on time. When I got it back I had an 'F' at the top. I was shocked and went to the teacher. He said another classmate had handed in a very similar paper obviously written by the same person. He just decided to fail us both because he did not know who had actually written it. I told him my rough draft had disappeared just a few days prior to the due date. I challenged him as to whose writing style he thought it might have been, taking into account the study habits of the other student. My grade was changed.

Grade nine was an interesting year. Over spring break a guy from Riverton torched our school. It was insulated with straw and burned really well. By the time the fire department got there the school was destroyed. By the end, the only thing indicating there had been a building was a basement full of ashes and other debris. Our spring break was a week longer than usual.

With that fire, all records were lost. There is no evidence anywhere that I completed Grades one to eight. The filing cabinet they were stored in was not fireproof, something that would now just not happen. We finished out the school year in the church with school supplies donated by Friesen Printers. By September, the new school was not entirely finished but finished enough to accommodate students. My Grade ten year was the first year I attended a school with a gym.

My final memories of my time in private school are not good ones. In gym class the other students thought it would be funny to pick on someone by aiming and trying to hit someone's legs with slap shots. I was the lucky student. This happened day after day. The teacher did nothing. There were days I could not stand up to get out of bed in the morning and I missed more than one day of school because of this. To this day, I have reminders of this as I still get severe leg cramps because of the scar tissue.

One thing I am thankful for is parents who stayed involved in my education, even though we attended a 'good' Christian school. The teacher I had for Grades eight to ten left me alone because of this I am sure. He was let go after that year because it was discovered by the board he was acting out sexually toward a number of girls and making extremely inappropriate comments to some male students. After the meeting with the board and some very concerned parents, he was allowed to finish out the year. I think that was a mistake. He should have been fired right then. Even if it meant there would have been a brief interruption of studies for the students in that room.

After the meeting, which Mom and Dad attended, Dad asked me why I had never mentioned to him what was going on in our class. I told him the teacher had never behaved to me in this way and I didn't feel it was my duty to tattle. I fully thought the other students were reporting it to their parents. I know now I should have told Dad as soon as I saw it once and not assume others were reporting it to their parents. It might have saved some of those families personal disillusionment with Christianity.

For Grades eleven and twelve, I went to the public school in town. This was a big adjustment. I made some new friends. None of them were very close but it made my time there not so lonely. There was a guy in my class who had lost both of his parents, his brother and sister and grandma in one accident. He was in the same accident but survived. It is interesting how one's spirit can connect with another when there has been a commonality. I got along with him really well.

There were a number of occasions I remember involving him. One was on a very cold winter December day and I had just come in from going into town. He was sitting on the metal fire-proof safe in the entrance and gazing out with a very sad look on his face. I didn't say much to him as I entered. I just commented on this being a difficult time of year. He just looked at me with tears in his eyes and agreed. I wasn't sure when the accident had happened but from the paper later that week I learned it had been the next week.

What a lousy Christmas for a boy who was in Grade three when the accident happened.

Then there was the time in the multi-purpose room when our class was working on a big project. I forget what the project was but I remember what I did to him. I was carrying a full glass of water for cleaning paint brushes. I came up behind him and when I realized he didn't know I was there, I was going to just put a drop or two of water on his head to scare him. Someone alerted him to my presence and he turned around. He saw what I was about to do and threatened if I did it he would never give me a ride in his brand new sports car. He had received his inheritance money when he turned eighteen and had bought a car with some of it.

Wrong threat — because he got the whole cup dumped on him and then I ran. Later he told me as soon as he had uttered the threat he knew it would not have the effect on me like it would have had on the other girls. He so badly needed a friend that didn't care he was a rich student but rather liked him for being him. One morning, I was in the English class when he came up behind me and scared the living daylights out of me, which is actually pretty hard to do. When I turned around he was close enough to kiss me. I told him I was going to get even yet, as the other students laughed themselves sick.

A few days later I had the chance in biology class when he was sitting on the end of a table and I was at the other end. I lifted the table and he went flying. He did manage to catch himself and looked back at me. I asked if we were now even and held out my hand. He smiled and said we were as we shook hands.

During English class we had to do a number of speeches. One of them was a demonstration speech. I made a friendship bracelet. At the end of the speech I asked if someone wanted it. Kevin said he would take it. When I was fastening it to his wrist I noticed his hands were slightly scarred and somewhat deformed and he seemed uncomfortable with it. I asked him if it had been from the accident and he said yes.

When our class played baseball we were always on the same team. He would play shortstop and I would play back catcher. Interesting mix but it worked. He was very athletic, and I was about as non-athletic as he was athletic. One time, he wanted to tag someone 'out' at home base and had thrown hard towards me and I caught it. This surprised everyone, including me. When anyone else threw me a ball, I was bound to miss it. From that time on, when we were trying to repeat that play they threw the ball to him first and he threw the ball to me. I do not recall ever missing a catch when he threw it regardless of how hard it came toward me.

When I was in Riverton I started loving gym class. I went from being the worst female player to one of the best. I was so used to co-ed that I had learned the secret of cross-checking the guys even though I was much smaller than them. When we played in Riverton the gym teacher had a rule that the boys could not touch the girls but the girls could touch the boys. This worked out very well in my favour until he changed the rule for me. I guess the guys had complained to him that I was too aggressive and was able to knock them over too easily.

There was one time I had a spare and was in the library when a group of students came in with an Ouija board. I knew about them but had never actually seen one. They started playing with it and a spiritual darkness came over the library. I started praying that the board would not work so they would lose interest in it. Then they asked it a question that had a rather straightforward answer — How many people are in this room? I knew instantly that the board would give them a wrong number because it would not recognize me. I was right. It gave them a number one short.

After trying to correct the board, the board insisted on that number. A number of the students got up disgusted and said that if the board couldn't even get a simple number correct it was useless and walked away. Praise the Lord for his creative ways of fighting the enemy.

A final, and one of my favourite memories I have of Riverton is the time I had most of my grade and multiple others believing I had a hangover from drinking too much at a wedding. I had a headache and someone asked me if it was because I had drunk too much over the weekend. I told them yes because that is the way I answer questions from the peanut gallery. Boy, did that rumour spread! I just went along with it every time I was approached about it.

Near the end of the day Kevin (a guy from my grade) came up to me and told me he didn't believe it. He asked me what I had to drink at the wedding and I said punch that wasn't spiked. Boy was everyone mad at me because they felt like such fools. They accused me of telling them a lie but they had to admit I had never actually said I had alcohol over the weekend but had just agreed with them, saying yes. I told them if they knew me well enough they would have known I was pulling their legs.

A month or two before I graduated from high school, I had no idea what I was going to do next. I thought of working because I knew I didn't have money for school but Mom and Dad felt quite strongly I should go to Bible school. I spent an afternoon praying about it as I had in front of me a number of brochures from different schools: Steinbach Bible College, Providence Bible College, Briercrest Bible College, and Prairie Bible College. By the end of the day, I had decided to apply to Prairie Bible College in Alberta.

This was the school Mom had been at when Dad and she had gotten engaged. Many people assumed I chose Prairie because Mom pressured me to do so. This was not true. In fact, most of my time spent with God that afternoon was spent trying to talk Him out of what I thought He was saying. Mom would not give me an answer when I asked for her input, she just told me to pray about it. It was a difficult decision because I was a home body and the thought of going out of the province was terrifying. I desperately wanted to stay close to home. Looking back, I can see how going to a Bible school close to home would not have been a wise decision on a number of levels.

Mom and Dad endorsed the decision and the application was sent off. I was accepted. Preparations began. Mom and Dad drove me to Alberta because Mom wanted to see her friends again. Just before we left Debbie and I were sure Mom was again pregnant. This made it that much harder to leave. Of course they didn't tell us as soon as they knew and that was a mistake. They should have known already that if they wanted to surprise us with the news of another pregnancy, they would have to get on it quickly. When my family got back to Manitoba Debbie told me Mom was pregnant. They finally told the ones at home and sent me a letter with the news. To their credit they immediately told us the due date. Debbie told them we already knew Mom was pregnant and we had calculated the due date as well. I love my parents but why on earth would they have thought we wouldn't figure it out? After all, we figured it out the second time already.

Chapter 5

I was a mess. I did not want to leave home but I had committed myself. We travelled to Alberta with our trusty mustard yellow Ford F-150 truck and Grandpa Reimer's truck camper on the back. The camper had not been used for a while. When we were packing it up, we started cooling off the fridge. I questioned the funny smell that was being emitted. They could faintly smell it but said it would go away once the fridge was fully cooled.

By supper time, I had a major headache and the smell was getting stronger all the time. I described it as the smell of a chicken barn. I was told I should quit complaining because no one else seemed to smell it anymore.

I almost didn't make it to Bible school. I went up to the bed above the cab to lay down because by now I was feeling outright sick. Not long after, I started having trouble breathing. Rebekah had joined me and I asked her to hit my back to help me breathe. After a bit even that wasn't helping.

Someone looked into the area and told her to stop hitting me. She said I had asked her to. The person just shrugged their shoulders and sat back down. Not long after, Rebekah must have realized something wasn't right and told the others that I was going to throw up. Dad stopped the camper and came to the back to open the door. He got there and I was still on the bed. He said to get out quickly and then realized it must be much worse than wanting to throw up. He hurried to the bed and helped me sit up and I passed out. He quickly got me out of the camper and realized I was barely breathing.

We were miles from anywhere and he did the first thing that came into his head. He started hitting me on the back rhythmically and prayed fervently. I started breathing easier once I had been out of the camper for a bit. When he asked me why I had not said anything. I told him I had been told to quite complaining because no one was taking me seriously about the smell. The fridge was immediately turned off and I then was put in the truck cab and the windows were rolled down.

It took days before I felt I didn't have congested lungs and breathing was normal. My back also had bruises on it from Dad hitting it but if he had not done that I am not sure I would have survived. Every time he hit he knocked the air out and I was able to get a fresh breath because my air pipe was almost closed.

The next day they took the camper to a shop and the mechanic told them there was a leaking pipe and the coolant vapour was being put into the air of the camper. Ironically, the vapour was almost smell less so I may not have actually been smelling it but the effect it was having on me was so much like what I experienced in the chicken barn that my mind was making me smell it. I was the first person to be affected but it would only have been a matter of time before everyone would have succumbed to its effects and it would have poisoned us all. It was a definite distraction from the pending separation.

We arrived at Prairie. The one good thing about all this is that when Mom had been dean of women there before she said yes to Dad, the school had matched her up with staff family to be her family while she worked there. They did this for any single staff member. The family Mom had been paired with was Abe and Martha Wiebe. They were still there and to top it off they had a daughter my age who was also starting her first year of Bible school. This made me feel slightly more at home as they extended to me the right to be 'part' of their family while I was there, just like Mom had been. I think this made Mom feel more at ease too. Then came the day they left. They said good-bye and I headed into the line to get my picture taken.

Whose brainwave was that anyway? When my turn in front of the camera came, my eyes were completely bloodshot from crying. I went to rinse my face with very cold water and tried to stop crying at least until the pictures were done. All things considered the picture didn't turn out that bad. My eyes were a little red but unless you had seen me immediately before or after the picture you would never know the truth. To top it off, my eyes were also still a little red from the poisoning on the way up so I blamed the redness on that.

No sooner was the picture taken than the water fountain started up again. I managed to make it through the first week but barely. I was overwhelmed with all the work that would need to be done in the semester and all the activities planned for that week. Being surrounded by so many people all the time was very hard for me. I needed down time because that is where I get my energy. Was I glad when the week was done! This first week of school for the next two years was not one that I ever looked forward to. I would have been happy to be excused from all the activities.

During the first week of classes we were given syllabi which included all the homework for each course. Even though I knew these were not all due immediately I freaked out. My Resident Assistant helped me out by sitting down with me and a day planner and charting out when the assignments were due. After that it seemed more doable. In this calendar I also put numbers on each day — day zero being the day I was going home for Christmas. Those numbers kept me going as I saw them get smaller.

In that first month, I got a letter from Dad telling me I would have another sibling. No surprise there. Debbie and I had already figured it out before we left home.

The first Thanksgiving weekend was the hardest. Mom later told me it was usually the 'hump weekend' of the semester for first-time students. For me it was, but not in the way that she had meant. That weekend was hard but it was hard for several reasons. I did miss being home and even though Grandma and Grandpa Wiebe took me with them for the weekend it wasn't the same. The other reason it was hard was because of what I was thinking about. I had hoped I would be successful in leaving my past behind me; this was a new start. That was not the way it seemed to be working out. I felt haunted by the insecurities and hurts of the past. I lost all hope and in my mind there was only one option. I was going to call it quits in life.

When someone commits suicide I now hurt for them. To most people it seems like such a selfish thing to do but unless you have been at the brink of taking your own life you have no idea how life without hope feels. When you lose hope, you lose your ability to feel and think about others. It is like the darkest night in your soul. It is just like the very essence of life is gone and you are in some ways already moving through life on auto-pilot.

I couldn't think of what my roommate would go through when she found me or how my family would feel as they got the news. In fact, there was little feeling at all in this state; it all became factual. I planned on overdosing and filling the room with the smell of ammonia. I knew with the ammonia my throat would close and knocking out myself with drugs would make the suffocating less of a struggle. A few days before I was going to carry out this bad mistake I made a comment to my psychology professor on the way out of the class.

The gist of the comment was that it would be nice if life worked like that, referring to something said in class. He stopped me and told me he wanted to meet with me in his office. What he heard in that statement I do not know but he saved a life that day. Right there, he pulled out his day planner and made an appointment. I now felt obligated to at least wait until the appointment was over and this annoyed me a little. The following week I showed up in his office and he told me outright that I was worth a lot in God's eyes and he would do everything in his power to stop me from killing myself.

He told me I needed to come for a counselling session every week and if I needed to, I could call him at any time of day or night. I was in shock because he had no way of knowing about my plans and that even one person cared was overwhelming for me because I didn't even know how to process that information. I had lost the ability to feel. This started a long journey back to emotional health. Looking back I realized why God had sent me to Prairie:

1. He knew I would need Don Masterson and he was on staff at Prairie Bible Institute.

2. God also knew that during this time of healing I needed to be far away from the insecurities that had hidden my problems because if I had been closer to home it would have been too easy to slip back to the status quo.

Now I had the time to become more established in the 'right' emotional pattern. There were two songs during my journey that were very comforting and encouraging. I listened to them often. To this day they bring tears to my eyes when I hear them.

The first one was 'Replace it with your love' by David Meece. It speaks about the process of letting God's love take out and replace all the hurt and bitterness in your life. The second song was 'I'm accepted' by DeGarmo and Key. This song speaks about my acceptance coming from God and not from the things, circumstances, or people that surround me.

Since then I have done for at least one person what Mr. Masterson did for me. I was talking with my young friend on the phone and as she was talking I sensed an underlying tone that I recognized all too well. I told her I would see her in the fall (this was spring) and she said I would. I repeated what I had said twice more and then she asked me what I meant. I told her she knew what I meant. I also told her life was worth living and it was okay to seek help from someone she trusted. That fall she asked me how I had known she had planned to take her life that summer. I told her I had been at that point and someone had pulled me back from the brink and I guessed that is why I was so sensitive to that despondent and hopeless spirit.

I started anticipating a call from home about mid-March. On the evening of March 21st, 1989 I got the call from the switchboard that I was to come to the administration building to take a call from Dad in five minutes. I got there in probably about two. As I waited, the switchboard personnel must have wondered what was going on as I paced the floor. The call came and I grabbed the phone before the first ring was done. It was Dad calling to tell me I had another sister but she had no name. Mom and he were wondering if I could give them some ideas in the next twenty-four hours. He had called me first and after he talked with me, he was going to call home.

Sadly, this time they had not hid it from Grandma Friesen. With a party line, she could pick up the phone and listen in every time it rang for our place. She did this for every call that evening and really ticked Debbie off. When Dad had called Grandma had been on the phone as well and he said this was good because then he didn't have to make two calls. Debbie just about hung up on him. I am not sure why they didn't follow the protocol of the previous time and just wait to tell the family when Dad got home.

Our Grandma Friesen could drive us nuts sometimes, but we truly love her. I have many good memories of time spent with her. I spent every other Thursday with her one year working on a quilt together. You can tell which part she quilted and which part I did. I missed her singing 'Happy Birthday' to me this year because she was in the hospital because of a blood clot. Other years she would often sing to me three times: the day before in case she couldn't get through on my birthday, on my birthday because it was my birthday, and the day after because she wasn't sure if she had remembered on my birthday. I (and my family) have also received many scarves, two quilts that she made herself, and two quilted baby blankets for our daughter. She is often heard to say that the thing that makes her happy is that the "family loves each other". Dispite her character flaws (of which we all have many) she has lead her family by example in this area. There is always room for one more and this is evident by the number of non-family members that are included in all our gatherings. Thanks Grandma for this heritage of love and acceptance of others.

I was so excited I told everyone I met that I had just had another baby sister. I do not know how many times others tried to correct me and said. "You mean a niece." My response was, "It was my mom that had the baby. I know what I'm talking about." After a bit though I started getting irritated with the people who said this — like I didn't know the difference between a sister and a niece. It was a hard month till school ended. I wanted to see her in person and hold her, not just see pictures. An interesting fact is that I am closer in age to Mom (seventeen years seven months) than I am to Rachel (eighteen years nine months).

I had started Bible school being registered in the two year program. When I came back the second year I switched it to a four year program. I never graduated with that diploma. The first semester of my third year I became quite sick, sick enough for the dean to deem it necessary for a trip to emergency which I took kicking and screaming. I spent twenty-four hours in emergency under observation. After all the blood work was back they had a diagnosis. My immune system was shutting down.

I have a few theories as to why. It could have been the environment I was living in. The dorm was full of substances I was allergic to, and all my stress could have aggravated that. Regardless of the reason it became obvious I would not be finishing the diploma. The doctor said I had two choices — leave school now or take a week away from school and recover a little so I could make it to the end of the semester. The dean was there as he gave me these two options. This was at the end of October, right before mid-terms.

I thought of leaving school right away but I was about two weeks past them being able to refund the semester. I decided with the dean's approval to take a break. She helped me work out a schedule with the professors to do the mid-terms a little late and give me an extension on the papers that were due at that time. I went to visit Charles and Karen Cox. They lived in Didsbury, about forty minutes from the school. Mom had gone to Bible school with Karen and they had remained good friends.

I had visited them on the occasional weekend already in my past two years at school. They graciously opened their home to me and I was able to have a week of rest and relaxation. I always looked forward to having butter on my bread when I visited them. That Christmas break I came home and never returned to finish what I had started. This was a hard thing for me but I realized God had had me there for that time and His purpose had been accomplished. I left an emotionally healthier person than when I had arrived.

Looking back, I would do Bible school a little differently next time. I would go and not look at a degree but at the courses I would like to take. I have thought of finishing my degree but by now I would have probably lost most of my credits because of the time that has lapsed and the courses I did take are so outdated. The truth is, I think God had me there not for the school itself but for what He wanted to do in me personally.

Chapter 6

From the time I left Bible school till December 1999 I rented living space from various relatives. This helped me as many of the jobs I had during that time were very low paying with few hours. In the fall of that year, Debbie and I started looking for a place of our own to rent. We found a sublet that was very reasonably priced and about two blocks from where I worked. It was a ground level unit on Grant Ave in Winnipeg. It was exciting for me — a space I could call my own. The caretakers were great and the people in the block were very quiet (no party animals) and we got to know probably half of the tenants during our stay there.

There were two tenants that stood out though. One was a man who was in the units only about half a year. He had just separated from his wife. We got to know each other better because we loaned him a cup of milk at about 10:30 p.m. one Saturday night. This led to a ride to work for me one day. He shared with me how he wished he and his wife could get back together. I told him we would pray for him as a family.

Two to three months later he met me in the parking lot and told me he was moving — back in with his wife. I did a dance right there in the parking lot and gave credit to God. At the end of the month when he was moving out, Mom and

Dad had come to visit and Dad met him in the hallway. He introduced himself and told him how glad we were that he and his wife were resolving things. Dad offered him a New Testament and he accepted it gladly. Dad told him if they kept it at the centre of their marriage, the marriage would work. He promised they would read it together often.

The other tenant was a black lady who lived above us. She was out here from Africa but had left her daughter behind with her mother while she got established. One morning Debbie came out of the apartment to see her being taken away by ambulance. She had fallen in the tub the night before and hadn't been able to get out. In the morning she had finally managed to get herself out to a phone and called a friend. The friend had come and called 911. The night before she had heard me in the bathroom a little and had tried to get my attention.

We realized then how soundproof the units were because I had not heard her. I remember thinking she must be having a bath because I could hear someone in the tub but the noise level or what I heard did not signal an emergency to me. I felt so bad. She had broken her hip and was in the hospital for a while and then came home with homecare till she was fully recovered.

During this time she asked Debbie and me to check up on her in the evenings and for me to unlock the door before I left for work in the morning so homecare could get in. She did not want to give homecare her key. For the next two months we did this for her as well as get her mail. We have seen her on occasion since then; her daughter has come to Canada and they are doing well. Her mother was going to move here as well but the cold of the first winter sent her packing for 'Home'.

Purchasing our first home was very unplanned and happened very suddenly; before Debbie and I knew what had taken place we owned a home together. Aunt Betty (the one we had lived with before the apartment) came over one Sunday evening for a visit. During the visit she asked us if we wanted to buy her place for the price she paid for it five years earlier. She was thinking of buying a place on the same bay that was being sold by Uncle Awln and Aunt Evelyn (her sister — another aunt). They had a three bedroom house and she had a two, and they also had a much bigger yard.

We all kind of laughed about it and nothing more was said. The next day Debbie told me she had not been able to sleep well the night before and we should really consider this. She had done the math and she figured it would be better for us financially than renting. I listened and that night I couldn't sleep. We approached Aunt Betty and she wasn't sure yet if she wanted to move. By Thursday, we had decided we would tell Uncle Awln and Aunt Evelyn we wanted to purchase their house. We already had an appointment at the bank for Friday.

When we called them they said Betty still hadn't gotten back to them but if she didn't want it they would work with us. When Aunt Betty heard we had expressed interest in their place, she quickly decided she would buy it. On Friday we went to the bank and were pre-approved for the mortgage. By the next Saturday we were sitting down and the papers were signed. Within two weeks we went from being renters without a thought of buying to having bought our own home.

We told our landlords and they didn't seemed overly unhappy about losing us as tenants. We did find someone to rent the place. They gave us back our damage deposit and signed a new rental agreement with the other tenants for a year. We realized why they had been so happy for us when we were informed in December that the building had been sold to a big company. When we had rented it was being run by a family. The company moved in and made major changes, then jacked up the rent to almost double what we had been paying.

Chapter 7

I had signed up with Candlelight Matchmakers in the spring of 2000. I was a little nervous about this. The agreement was for a year's duration, or for meeting with six potential matches. I met my sixth match in 2004. I was very unhappy with the 'Christian men' she said she had so many of. I saw many profiles I turned down immediately because they either drank occasionally or were divorced. I spoke with quite a number and after the first conversation I knew I was not interested. Of the six I agreed to meet, only three did I meet more than once. I was actually relieved when the sixth one came and went.

About a year later, Diane called me up and asked if she could send me a few more profiles. I made it clear I was not renewing my membership but she said it didn't matter. I guess she was not used to not having success within the first "year".

The first one she sent me I met with probably about six times and by the end it was apparent to both of us that it was not a match. She sent me a few more I didn't even bother meeting. In January of 2006 she called me and asked if I would consider looking at one more profile. I told her she was free to send it but it was a waste of her time. Apparently,

Rob had told her the same thing. He was as turned off with the 'Christian women' she had sent as I was with the men. I got the profile and looked it over. I wasn't really impressed but I wasn't really turned off either.

I told her I would consider talking to him if he wanted to talk to me. Apparently he said he would talk to me because a time was arranged for me to call him. The reason I was going to call him was because I had one sister living with me who did not know I was signed up with a matchmaker and I didn't want her to find out. Later he told me he was sure that earlier on he had been sent my profile but had declined because of the fact that I said one of the things I would not like in a spouse was that they would watch a lot of TV. He watched a lot of TV (and still does).

As luck would have it, the Friday evening for the arranged call a movie night was planned at our house with a few sisters. I was not too concerned because I thought the phone call would not be very long. The phone call lasted longer than I had thought it would — about thirty minutes. During this call I brought up every topic I could where I thought there might be a conflict of interest, ranging from finances to how many children he wanted. I got off the phone and went and enjoyed the party. I was sure I wouldn't hear from him again.

He called me Monday as we had pre-arranged. I was thinking he would call and tell me he didn't think it would work. Was I ever mistaken. It seemed God had already prepared him for this phone call over a year previously when my cousin Shelly and her husband Jake, who attended his church, had approached him about possibly meeting their cousin. This had never happened but they had been praying for us since and had asked God to bring us together if it was meant to be.

All that weekend Rob had been thinking about our conversation and had thought there was something familiar about me. It dawned on him when he walked up to the church doors that Sunday that this was the girl Shelly and Jake had talked to him about a year previous. After the church service he approached Jake and asked him a few questions to confirm his suspicions. In the meantime Shelly had joined them and when he told them he had just "talked to her" they were in shock. When he told me this on Monday night I was very confused. This was supposed to be the "it's not going to work out" call and now this. Now what?

It was a short call after which I called Shelly and told her to promise that no one would hear about this. She of course wanted to know how on earth this had taken place and I told her about signing up with Candlelight Matchmakers years before. She said they would continue to pray and would not tell a soul. This started a battle raging in my spirit that would not stop until August. During this time I started journaling (something that is not easy for me) because I hoped it would bring clarity to my mind and put into perspective what was happening.

During every call that followed I tried to find a reason to call it off but I just couldn't. This was unusual because I had had no trouble doing this all the other times. We met for the first time at Tim Horton's on March 27th. Debbie had to go somewhere so she dropped me off and did her thing. The arrangement was that we would meet up again close to home and I would come home with her as if nothing else had happened. Remember the sister that was living with us that knew nothing about this?

I chose not to get dressed up or do anything with my hair or make-up thinking he would not be impressed. This didn't work out as planned. Apparently he was not to be scared off easily. I would have to try harder. On Easter of that year he went to visit his parents and brought me back a box of chocolates from Bernard Callebaut (a high end chocolate shop where his mother worked). He dropped them off at our house. I met him outside because Judith was inside. I said a friend was stopping by to see me. When I came in with a box of chocolates, she didn't ask any questions.

I am not sure when he told his parents he was 'talking' to someone but my parents didn't find out until the end of April that I was 'talking' with a potential mate. When I told them they were a little surprised that I had not told them sooner. I told them I had not mentioned it to them because I was sure it would not work out and I was scared Dad would try to 'help' the situation. Dad had the idea from the Basic Life Institute, which teaches a woman is under her dad's authority until she is married, and that he had some role in this area of my life. In my opinion this idea could be taken too far. I was already thirty-five years old and had lived on my own for many years. The idea that a father should be heavily involved with a thirty-five-year-old woman's courtship seemed a little ludicrous to me. However I highly valued his opinion in the matter.

There comes a time when a father and mother need to trust their children to make mature choices, especially when they have lived on their own for over fifteen years. I told Dad I respected his input and advice but I was no longer under his roof. My family met him on the May long weekend of that year. I had hoped only my immediate family would meet him but it was not to be. Uncle Ruben drove by, saw his Grand Prix there and had to drive in to see who the driver of the car was. I knew the secret was out. It was somewhat awkward because I was still trying to find a way to call it off, but it seemed he got along well with my family.

The next weekend I met his parents and family. We met with his parents and an uncle and aunt in Morden before a cousin's wedding. The meeting went well but I was very nervous. On the way home that night we had a conversation about kissing. He was the one to bring it up and I was shocked at what he said. He said he wanted the first kiss to be at his wedding. I told him that was my desire as well. At that point I almost up and kissed him because I could not believe I had actually found someone who had the same desire. I was so grateful for this because I now knew I would not have to be the one to put on the brakes in the physical part of our relationship.

The day before I met his parents, I must have been a bit more uptight at work than usual and people did notice. They asked me if there was something wrong. There was no way I was going to say anything to them at this point. I surely wouldn't take any counsel from them and they didn't need to know yet. All but one of them didn't know anything till I was engaged. Mid-August I did tell my supervisor (who I had a really good relationship with) about him and told her that the Friday back in May when I had been somewhat distracted and preoccupied was the day before I met his family. My co-workers did not know about the relationship until we were engaged. When I announced our engagement, one of the first questions I got was, "When is the baby due?" I told them I was not pregnant and that we hadn't even kissed yet. No one believed me when I said we had never kissed and a few were still sure that I was pregnant.

On June 2nd he came out for pizza night with Jake and Shelly. He asked me if we could go for a walk. I agreed, not sure what to expect. He gave me birthday presents and asked me if he could court me with the intent of marriage. The birthday presents were an ankle bracelet and a birthday book for us to write a message to each other on our birthday every year. He apparently thought he had found his bride. I wasn't so sure but I said yes. The only reason I said yes was because I knew I would still be able to call it off if I found out something that would warrant it.

A week or two after we started going out we had a more in depth talk in his car outside his place about the physical part of our relationship. This was good and I would encourage all new 'couples' to be intentional about this part of the relationship. He told me he would also like to stay away from frontal hugs as a friend had told him that had been a source of great temptation in his relationship. I fully agreed. We did not kiss or have a frontal hug until we were pronounced husband and wife.

The idea was that we would get to know each other on an intellectual and emotional level to make sure we wanted to get married. On his birthday I drove to Steinbach with a picnic supper and we found a quiet place in the park to eat it. It was a good evening. The following weekend we went to the Red River Ex. It was there on a swing ride that we held hands for the first time other than when we prayed at meals with my family.

Over the summer we talked on the phone a lot and got together occasionally. My summer was busy because Debbie was gone with the Navy and I was doing Mom and Dad's books for their business Integrity Foods. I went out every week-end to help with pizza nights as well. I also spent a week at camp as head cook again. On August 11th we attended his roommate's wedding. This was our first public appearance together. August 11th was a turning point in my spirit. We had originally planned I would meet him in Steinbach but he got off work early and I got off late so he came to the city to pick me up to save time. The route from Steinbach was more direct but when we went from Winnipeg we took a slightly different route and the time difference was less than me getting to Steinbach and both going from there.

He showed up at my door with flowers. Years earlier I had asked God to give me a sign that the man was the right one. I had asked God that he would give me seven red roses. Rob had brought me seven red roses! I could no longer entertain the idea that this was not to be. He apologized because he had only meant there to be six roses, being symbolic of the six month mark in our friendship. He said he had no idea how the seventh rose got in there. He remembered the florist pulling out six roses and then putting one to the side because she did not like the way it sat in the arrangement and getting one more. On the way to the city he had looked over and recounted the roses and there were seven.

After a couple of recounts he had thought of taking the extra one out but decided to leave it in. By this time I had done a number of recounts myself and told God I was now ready to move ahead toward marriage in this relationship. I accepted Rob's apology but did not tell him till the end of the weekend why the seven roses were so significant and the implications if he had removed the extra rose. Right at that moment I was so choked up I was not able to communicate this to him.

We went to his roommate's wedding on a Friday night. We spent the night in Steinbach and came to the city in the morning for my friend's wedding. This was the first any of them had seen or heard of Rob. One of the ladies in our worship team was always talking about how she could spot a girl who was going out. She was one of those that could get on your nerves.

I had determined they would not find out about Rob till I was good and ready to introduce him. I think I almost gave a few of the worship team members' heart attacks when I walked into the wedding with him. The lady who had been so arrogant about the whole issue told me she had suspected something for a bit already. When I asked her for how long she said for about a month or a month and a half. When I told her it had been for a little over six months already, she back-peddled and said she had never said that at all.

After the wedding, we headed to my parents' place for pizza night. On the way up Rob told me for the first time verbally he loved me. It was on the stretch of the number eight highway close to Misty Lake Lodge. On the way back to Winnipeg on Sunday on the same stretch of road I told him about the significance of the seventh rose. Now it was his turn to be shocked.

Chapter 8

Rebekah had come home for a visit. Debbie, Judith, Rebekah and I were headed out of the city for the weekend. Rob was going to once again join our family. This was the first time he would meet Rebekah. We were going to head out of the city right after lunch on September 8th, but we were delayed because we decided to visit someone in the hospital. We had just turned onto McPhilips Street when Debbie looked in the rear view mirror and said she was sure Rob was right behind us. As it turned out our slight delay and his getting off work early caused us to meet. I switched cars at the 7-Eleven and both cars continued on to Riverton.

We stopped for gas at the Shell station half way between my parents place and Winnipeg. After fuelling up and a bathroom break we were on our way again but Rob stopped before we had left the parking lot. He turned to me and asked me if I would marry him as he handed me a box. I was taken completely off guard. I was expecting him to propose the following weekend, because then his parents were going to be at Mom and Dad's. He had actually planned to propose later that evening because he had not anticipated meeting me along the way. He had just not been able to wait till we got there.

I think I said yes three times, the first two being whispered. He told me he had asked Dad the previous weekend if he had their permission to ask me to marry him and Dad had said yes. I remember Rob driving a bike off the yard with Dad to go check up on the neighbours' cows while the neighbours were away. I remember the thought crossing my mind wondering if he might be doing that but I didn't give it a second thought until he told me in the car.

I thought that had been a very considerate and respectful thing for him to do. In some ways though I think it was a formality because the truth was we were both in our mid-thirties and Dad and Mom would have said yes because they trusted me. I had been on my own for many years and valued their opinion from early on in the relationship. If at any point they had expressed serious doubt, I would have been more than willing to break it off.

We caught up with the others in Riverton because Mom had asked me to pick up the mail and I wasn't sure the others would remember. Rob got out of the car as well and he and Rebekah met for the first time on Main Street in Riverton. We did not announce our engagement to them there. The first thing I did when we reached my parents farm was to go find Debbie. She was downstairs and I told her I was engaged. She was excited but not overly surprised. I went out to find Mom and Dad and the others and told them next. I wasn't much help that pizza night.

We spent a fair bit of time on the phone that night as we called his family and others we wanted to tell personally. By the end of the evening we had also decided which weekend we were planning to have the wedding (November 25/26). It took a week or two to decide on whether to have it on the Saturday or the Sunday. We chose Saturday based on which venues were available for what we knew was going to be a very large wedding.

Our initial guest list was a little over seven hundred people. This was cut down to three hundred and twenty by the last cut. Our final count for who showed up was between two hundred and eighty and three hundred. We based this on how full the church was as many people did not sign the guest pages.

In the span of eleven weeks we were engaged, planned a wedding and bought a house. Needless to say it was a busy eleven weeks! When my church in Winnipeg announced our engagement there was another engagement announced. Curtis announced the other engagement first and then ours — their wedding was to take place in about two years and we were going to be married in nine weeks. We became engaged on the same weekend.

When I heard his announcement I thought we were crazy because all I could think about was what all needed to get done yet. We found out that others thought so too, after the service when they came to congratulate us. Many of them were unaware I was even going out with someone.

I found a white dress on the rack which I liked, which was a good thing because there was no way there was time for a custom order. A few alterations were needed to change the straps from a halter fit on the top to straps that criss-crossed on the back and it was ready. It was a fairly simple dress with some beading that had a fitted bodice with an A-line skirt, but it had a touch of elegance. It was in reality a grad dress but was in stock and fit me perfectly in the bodice.

Our venues were booked. We had to have the ceremony and the reception in different places. I had hoped to find a venue able to hold them both but to no avail. Many of the larger places were booked with Christmas parties already. In hindsight I would do that differently.

We would have had it at the Fort Garry Hotel on Sunday. The reason I steered away from that idea was because I would have needed to get RSVPs and the timeframe was very short. If we had had it there, they would have done the decorating and the meal and the total cost of the wedding would not have been significantly greater than what we did. Our decorations were limited because of the timeframe. The reception area was more decorated than the church. The food prep was a significant part of the work.

We were going to have dainties and fruit and veggie platters. Mom thought this was not going to be enough. She added dips, crackers, cheese, meat, etc. and before we knew it we were serving a full out meal when the invites had said a light lunch. This brought our cost up significantly.

The flowers were ordered. We had three attendants each. I asked my attendants to pick the colour they wanted for their dresses. I figured they would be wearing them so I wanted them to like the colour and style so they could wear them again. It also was good for me because then I would not have to make those decisions. They decided to go with black and they all choose dress styles they liked. I then decided they would carry three red long stemmed roses tied together with a silver ribbon, while I carried seven red long stemmed roses. They bought their dresses and we bought the silver necklaces to go with their outfits.

Rob wore a black suit with a white shirt and a silver tie. The guys then wore black dress pants with a white shirt (no jacket). We purchased their ties, which were mostly a silver grey with some darker accents. We decided that if the guys wore black suit jackets as well that everything would be too black.

A few weeks before the wedding, I took my purity ring to the jewellers to have it enlarged to fit Rob's ring finger. It was to be his wedding band.

Our mutual friend (my cousin's husband), Jake was our MC for the reception. We met with him and Shelly to discuss what his role would look like. The one thing I remember about the evening was that I asked Jake very specifically to treat Debbie like a true lady that day. I knew it would be a hard day for her. He promised to do that for me. True to his word, the day of the wedding he 'loved' on Debbie. I don't think he spent much time with Shelly that day.

The rehearsal went well. Last minute instructions were given, and ties were tied for the groomsmen that did not know how to tie them. We retired for a good night's sleep. HA HA! I didn't sleep much that night. Debbie and I talked and cried a lot that evening/night. I remember wondering if I was actually doing the right thing. I had so hoped Debbie would get married first because I figured I would be better off without her than she would be without me. I knew she depended on me a lot.

On November 25th my day began at 5:30 a.m. I knew there were some things that I had not finished, but it was too late now. Before Rob arrived a lot had to be done. There was the hair and make-up for me and my three attendants. The cat needed to be groomed once more. Hamburgers needed to be made for the honeymoon. And then the final step was getting into the dress. This is when I started getting nervous. I hoped that Rob would like the dress. When Rob saw me, his eyes teared up and he came to me as I stood at the bottom of the stairs. I was glad he loved my dress choice.

We headed out for pictures at the Manitoba Legislature building first. The day before was above freezing and we would have been able to have some pictures outside without freezing the flowers. Overnight it turned cold. The morning of the wedding it was cold and a little windy. This tempera-ture change also created some ice, so we had to walk carefully. We were about fifteen minutes late starting with the pictures. The pictures went okay. We got enough good pictures, so I could make a nice wedding album.

There were some good pictures but some basic things were missed, such as how my shawl looked (I had it buttoned up on the back of the dress). Many of the pictures were out of focus and there was not many of the wedding party because the wedding party was all over the place doing their own thing. I was continually corralling them in. I was stressed during picture taking because I felt I was the only one coming up with ideas and I do not think that it's the bride's job to keep people together and focused on the task at hand, during the photography sessions.

When the family left for the church to do the final set up there, they did not take the flowers along. Other than the flowers for decorating and the corsages not making it to the church, the ceremony went off without a hitch.

My beloved Aunt Katherine and Uncle Dave were both able to attend our wedding. My cousin who worked at the home and some of his children told me Uncle Dave could talk about nothing for a few weeks before that date other than coming to our wedding. The week before he had not been doing so well but they brought him anyway because he said they had to. I had confirmed with the ushers that they would be brought to the very front of the church. When I walked up the aisle, I saw him and I was so glad he had made it. Out of all my guests, I would have been most disappointed if they had not come to my wedding. It probably would have been almost enough to ruin my day.

After the ceremony, Mel and Janice had asked them if they wanted to go home now, but they were at the reception till the end. I was told later it had taken almost a week for him to fully recuperate physically, but all he could talk about was the wedding.

The church was full, so that means that there were about two hundred and ninety people at the ceremony. This was not reflected in the guest book signatures. We already had two places to sign because we knew there would be a lot of guests. Our guest book has the attendance at under two hundred people. This also disappointed me because I didn't think that we have to have an usher to make sure that the people signed. After all, isn't there a guest book signing at every wedding?

We did not have a long ceremony because we were getting married, not having a full church service. After we had said our vows, the pastor said, "Rob, you may now kiss your bride." This was the first time our lips met. What a rush of emotion. We had refrained from kissing since we met, but the temptation sure was present. After we had walked out of the sanctuary, we shared our first frontal hug in the lobby. Again, the emotions that surfaced were almost overwhelming and at the same time so exhilarating. By refraining from both of these activities until we got married, we saved our selves a lot of unnecessarily temptation in this area. It was easier not to feel those strong emotions that come with kissing and hugging when we knew that we saving sex till marriage.

Both of us had a surprise for the other during the ceremony. We had individually gone to the officiating pastor and arranged the surprises. Rob's surprise to me was a trumpet solo. I did not know that he played trumpet. The ring was my surprise to him. Before we exchanged rings, Uncle Al (Dad's brother) who was officiating the wedding told Rob and the audience about the ring that I was going to give Rob. He told how I had bought the ring 11 years ago and had used it for 11 years waiting to give it to the man who would become my husband. He said that as I put this ring on his finger that I was giving myself to him in my entirety — that emotionally and physically I had saved myself for him. Rob had a tear roll down his cheek, when he heard this and as I was placing the ring on his finger. This almost started me crying which would have ruined my make-up.

We had asked my Uncle Dwight (Aunt Lorna's husband) to write a song for our wedding. He agreed to do this. In his song he had include the symbols of seven red roses (he knew the significance of that) and the ring (but was unaware of the significance of that) for when we had doubts and hard times. Later he told me he had been pleasantly surprised when we had exchanged rings to hear the story of Rob's ring and realized how perfect the song actually was for our circumstances.

We arrived at the reception at the scheduled time. We had a good time with our family and friends. There was lots of visiting and picture taking. We earned enough money kissing to pay for our first night at the Hotel Fort Garry. For the record you do not need practice kissing, it comes quite naturally.

The thing I had feared happened with the food though. We had hired someone to look after the food table so Mom would not be tied up with that all evening. As it was, Mom did more than the person we had paid.

All the challenges aside, the program part of the reception went well. The people that shared were very encouraging and used great tact when it came to things they shared, with the exception of my dad who once again had to talk about Mommy (with Mom standing beside him). I had asked him not mention her but I guess he does it so often he did it out of habit. The whole wedding was videoed by my Uncle Awln.

After the reception, the core group (immediate families, the wedding party, people who had taken part in the ceremony, and all their spouses) went out for supper to Tony Roma's. We had ordered thirty identical plates, which consisted of two marinated grilled chicken breasts, baked potato and broccoli. We choose to have all the toppings for the baked potatoes on the tables instead of on the individual plates, because this was easier for serving and then there was also a lot more toppings for everyone. Everyone could order a drink of their choice. When we got there and I was doing a head count it appeared

I had ordered food for everyone but us. Not a problem. They just quickly brought in a small table and made up two more identical dishes. By seven, we wrapped it up and headed for the hotel.

If we had known on that night how hard the married journey would be I am not sure we would have signed up. Here we were, two older adults both well established in our habits and ideas working to create unity in one household. Throw in with this, external circumstances we had no control over and the years that followed appeared to be a bit of a gong show sometimes. I am thankful we have had God as the glue in the centre of the marriage or we would have been in trouble many times.

Chapter 9

February 22, 2007 — First miscarriage
Kipp: from the pointed hill, near to the heart of God

I found out on February 21st, 2007 one day before the completion of the miscarriage that I was actually pregnant. At the end of January I had gone to give blood and my iron had been low. I had just had my menstrual cycle a week before although it had seemed a little abnormal. I found out later that a miscarriage can take a month or two to complete. I was at work on February 22nd between my morning break and lunch when I started having what felt like severe period cramping. I hurried to the bathroom and got there before I miscarried. I knew this was the case because of the extreme blood loss, the clumps of what appeared to be uterine lining and cramping.

After resting for a few minutes I headed downstairs with a very heavy heart, not saying a word to anyone. I finished working the day and went to my hairdressing appointment. When I got home that night, I cried the evening away. Little did I know this would happen seven more times. I went to bed early that night and determined if I was rested in the morning I would head to work and that is what I did. By mid morning I realized that this had probably not been a wise idea. I did finish out the day but I told Karen (my supervisor) I had miscarried the previous morning and I would probably take the next two days off to recover.

I guess I was not aware of how much blood I had lost; it would take a while for my energy to come back. I mourned the loss of Kipp very deeply, which kind of surprised me because I had only known one day I was even pregnant. I know now that a loss of life at any stage is a loss of life. It needs to be mourned so there can be a going forward. Kipp is in heaven and one day we will meet him because he had a soul which made him fully human even though we could not yet see his formed body. We had no idea whether I had been carrying a boy or girl, but in order for us to put a face to the baby we lost we were advised a name would help give the baby an identity. This was the case for every child we lost. We chose names because of what they meant, not because we knew their gender.

I had my monthly cycle once in March and on April 22nd my period was a week overdue. I had been feeling a little nauseous for a few days and certain foods were giving me indigestion. My breasts were also feeling very tender. We did the test on a Sunday morning and were overjoyed when we saw a very clear plus sign before the test was actually considered complete. My seven months of all day sickness had started. I was sick the first five months and then again for the last two months. I thought I had awhile to order maternity wear for work, but two weeks later about two days after I had ordered the clothes, I had to approach the supervisor about the possibility of using sweats till the new pants arrived. I could no longer close the uniform. So much for not showing for the first three months. During these couple of weeks between finding out and starting to show, I was asked by Vince (guy in charge of gun training at work) if I was available for doing the gun training in June to get my personal firearms license. I was working at Brinks during this time. I was next on the list for the training as the lady senior to me had failed the course twice and now had to wait for another year before trying again. I didn't exactly want to tell him yet but my look said what I didn't verbalize.

There were two other people who figured out I was pregnant. One was my supervisor, who asked me if I was pregnant about four days after conception. I told her I didn't know. When the test came back, I told her she had been right but not to tell anyone yet. The other was a lady who drove one of the trucks. She approached me in the garage one day and asked me. I confirmed her guess, but again told her this was not public knowledge yet.

I gained over twelve pounds in the first trimester. By three months I was obviously pregnant. Thankfully, this is the one time we did not have to tell people I had miscarried. It was not until about three years later that we realized what a miracle this was.

I had morning sickness for seven to eight months of the pregnancy. My two months of reprieve came during the fifth and sixth month. November twenty-ninth was a glorious day. I remember walking over to the garbage can after I was ready to go home and throwing away the runners I had used at work. They were worn out and I had no intention of returning to work after maternity leave.

This was the day I had looked forward to for many years. I am not one of those women who felt a need to keep my job. I would rather be at home raising the family that God gave me than letting them be raised by the system. I had worked in a daycare in the past and knew that if that is where my children would end up I would choose to not have any. It would be cheaper and less hassle.

Chapter 10

December 31, 2007 — our only daughter
Tirzah: Pleasant, gentle
Deena: from the valley, peaceful
Reanne: gracious, gentle

During the month of December I had a project I wanted to get done. I had not yet put together our wedding album and knew once the baby came that this would be much harder to do. It was the type of project that needed a large window of time to focus without interruption. This idea was almost benched when on December 2nd I thought my water might be leaking and the Braxton-Hicks became consistent and stronger. After going to the hospital and being checked out, they said that I was not in labour and that I should go home and relax. By Christmas I had completed the album and done a major house cleaning.

The baby was due December 24th. This made our Christmas interesting to say the least. There were so many things going on and I could commit to none of them. We did make it to both immediate family gatherings though. On the twenty-sixth we had the gathering at my parents place in Riverton. The Wiebe gathering had taken place a few days previous. The next morning at about 4:00 a.m. we headed in to Winnipeg because I had started having contractions that were consistently regular. It turned out that it was pre-mature labour and they stopped sometime that afternoon.

I was tired of sitting around at home wondering when this baby would arrive, so we went to a Hildebrand gathering on December 30th. After a long afternoon, during which I was having Braxton hicks, we headed home. On the way home, my Braxton Hicks became quite strong but this was not so unusual because they had been like this frequently in the last month. We got home and got ready for bed.

At 9:45 p.m. we were just finished praying when I felt something very strange. It felt like my bladder had burst. I didn't know it was possible for a woman that pregnant to move that fast. I jumped out of bed and made it to the bathroom before my water burst entirely. All Rob heard from the bedroom was "uh-oh" and then the gush of water. He instantly realized that his night was just beginning. We knew we had to go to the hospital immediately because there was meconium in the fluid. This meant our baby had already pooped.

I tried to get dressed but the water kept coming. Finally, I just put my pants on and grabbed a towel. My contractions were about one and a half to two minutes apart. They continued like this, but without progressing until I received Pitocin. By the time we got to the hospital I was soaked down to the ankles. As I stood in the lobby waiting for Rob to park the car (the walk would have been good for me but it would have been a little chilly being so wet), a few people walked through the door and I got a few strange looks that turned to the "ooooh" sort of looks.

When we got to triage there was a couple ahead of us. The nurse said to go wait in the waiting room and called for another nurse to get me a pad to sit on. The nurse came out, took one look and told me to follow her. I was taken to a bed immediately and the triage nurse came in a little later to check me in. As I went in I apologised to the couple sitting there and they quickly assured me it was no problem. The look on their faces was interesting. It almost looked like they were reconsidering delivering their baby.

Because of the meconium, I was told if I had not delivered in twenty-four hours a C-section would be done. I spent the next three hours walking around the hospital. What a waste of time. I was no more dilated than when I had come in. At this time I sent Rob home to get some sleep because I knew I would need him more a little later than I did now. When they transferred me to the high risk area, I was assigned a nurse who was there at my beck and call. She stayed with me until Rob arrived.

I had not progressed any by six o'clock, so they put me on Pitocin. This did speed things up but it also was more painful because now the contractions were about a half to one minute apart with very little time if any to prepare for the next contraction. When Rob arrived at about seven o'clock the nurse gave him some pointers and stepped outside the room but was outside the door the whole time. She came in to check on me occasionally, when Rob called her in to ask her a question, or when Rob needed a break she came in and stayed with me till he came back. Around eight o'clock Dr. Gabriel came in (she happened to be on call) to see how I was doing. She knew I did not want to be drugged, so she made a few suggestions.

I did at that time take a shot of morphine so I could rest a bit between the close contractions. The morphine did dull the pain somewhat and it was the reprieve I needed. A little before lunch I got laughing gas. I'm not sure it really dulled the pain at all but it did give me a focus and because I could hear myself breathing I was able to slow breathe through entire labour.

Rob was a great support. When the contractions would come I would focus on his face and together we would breathe another contraction away. He told me again and again that I was doing a good job. At about three o'clock the contractions stopped. After a check by the nurse, the doctor was called. I had hoped to have Dr. Gabriel deliver the baby but she was off call at three o'clock. There was about a five minute break from any activity. I threw up, then the pushing started. The pushing lasted about one hour and fifteen minutes. It did not seem that long.

I had an intern doing the delivery. They asked me if it was okay and at that point I didn't care who did it. They also had an entire team of pediatric specialists in the room because she had pooped before she was born. The going was slow as the baby moved forward three steps and back two. I was not drugged so I could work together with my body and I did not rip at all.

When they told me she had crowned I asked if she had hair. This was more important to me than if she had all her fingers and toes. They probably had never heard that question before. They checked for me and said she did. I then got Rob to check and he confirmed, which he did reluctantly. When the head came out, I heard the intern talk through what she was doing. When she checked for the umbilical cord around the neck, she stated it was and that she would now slip it off. After a moment's pause I heard her tell the doctor that it seemed to tighten when she tried. The doctor immediately took over and after trying the same thing, she told me I needed to push out the baby right away, even before the next urge to push. It wasn't hard and as our daughter came into this world, I leaned back and took a deep breath.

I was unaware of the drama that then unfolded. Rob told me later he had looked on with shock as the doctor unwound the cord from her neck three times, counting each one. As soon as the cord was removed from her neck she hollered up a storm at her indignation of this turn of events. What a precious sound.

Rob had a very different set of emotions during labour and delivery. He told me later that he had felt so helpless with me being in so much pain and he couldn't do anything about it. When I had started throwing up just before the pushing started, I remember him saying that he was sorry that he had fed me the few spoons of soup and Jello earlier. The nurse quickly assured him that this happened quite often between the regular labour and the pushing.

The shock factor of the cord around her neck never hit me because I was so exhausted and relieved that the labour was over. By the time I would have cared, I already knew she was alright. For Rob however it seemed like a very long few seconds as he counted with the doctor. As she started crying he was very relieved.

I had to ask whether I had had a girl or a boy, because the medical staff was occupied with the unexpected emergency. They told me that I had a girl and I will never forget calling her by her name for the first time, "We have a Tirzah." Rob was asked if he wanted to cut the cord, which he did and she was hurried to the warming table. She weighed in at 3.175 kg (7 lbs) and 53.5 cm (21") long. And yes, she had a fair amount of hair.

The doctor was upset that a C-section had not been done because she had surely been in distress during the labour. She personally looked through the readout from the monitoring machine and was mystified that there was indeed no distress at any time during the labour. Despite the fact that she had pooped before she was born and had the cord around her neck three times, she was born with an Apgar score of 8.5, which is normal for a labor with no complications.

Rob was the first to hold her and I remember thinking, she already has her daddy wrapped around her little finger. After what seemed like an eternity, he brought her to me and put her in my arms. There were tears in his eyes. She looked up at me with such clear eyes. We couldn't take our eyes off each other. Before we left the delivery room, Rob told me that I never needed to do this again if I didn't want too. My response, "Give me a good nights' sleep and we can start over."

Breastfeeding came naturally for Tirzah. The nurse was going to show me how to do it and Tirzah latched on before I was even in 'the right position'. The nurse witnessed this and told me I would have no trouble in this department. Shortly after this we were moved to our room.

Later Rob told me that leaving the hospital that night had been one of the hardest things he had ever done. He felt he was leaving us unprotected. The male's need to protect came in strong the moment he first laid eyes on her. The emotions of delivering ended for me when Tirzah was born, but for Rob they lasted much longer and he told me the next day that he still felt like he was in some emotional turmoil. He was amazed at how quickly the emotions disappeared for me.

God had his hand on our little daughter. Only later would we discover how much of a miracle she was. She was healthy and very much alive, the very thing we had hoped for. We both felt like the labour, delivery and holding her for the first time was an extremely spiritual and emotional experience. How blessed I was to share this experience with my husband.

In the beginning of December we visited Uncle Dave and Aunt Katherine when I was nine months pregnant. Both of them were so excited for us and Aunt Katherine said to make sure to we let them know when the baby arrived and she could barely wait to hold the little one. Her health had been deteriorating over the previous couple of months.

After Tirzah was born, I got Rob to call Carl and Luella when he got home from the hospital. I wanted to make sure Uncle Dave and Aunt Katherine were told as soon as possible that we had had a little girl and we would be visiting soon. Rob was told that Aunt Katherine was not doing well and they didn't know how long she had. When we got home on January 2nd, 2008, we were making plans to head to Steinbach within the week so that Uncle Dave and Aunt Katherine could see her. We had been home for about four hours when we got the news that Aunt Katherine had gone to her eternal home. I cried.

Luella told me later that they had told her about Tirzah and the only thing she could talk about in her last day or two was to ask when we were coming. I think that if I had known this, we would have left the hospital earlier and gone directly to Steinbach. Dad, Debbie, Tirzah and I went to the funeral. Tirzah was exactly one week old. We were invited to stay for the family time after the funeral, which came as no surprise. As we were saying good-bye to everyone, Uncle Dave wanted to hold Tirzah one more time. With more aggression than was necessary, he pushed his still half full plate across the table and indicated that he wanted to hold Tirzah again. There was not a dry eye around the table as he held her.

Because of Parkinson's, Uncle Dave had excessive amounts of saliva. He held her ever so tightly and they both gazed intently into each other's eyes no more than a foot from each other. As he held her his drool soaked her blanket but I didn't care. I knew we were witnessing a bonding of spirits and everyone around the table could feel it. After what seemed like an eternity he handed her back and said I had better take care of his little girl and I was to bring her to visit often.

We visited as often as we could although I feel it was not often enough. When we came to visit, the nurses often asked him if it was his great-grandchild. Sometimes we would correct them and sometimes we wouldn't. He loved her. He kept every picture we gave him of her on his wall. When we were contacted on January 3rd, 2011 that he was on his way home to Heaven, we changed all our plans and headed straight to Steinbach to say our goodbyes. He was already for the most part unresponsive, but he did acknowledge our presence. I held his hand for a while. He lived much longer than first anticipated but on January 5th, 2011 he passed away, never really regaining consciousness. Rob took the day off for his funeral. After the funeral we once again joined the family for the evening. What a blessed time. It seems that no matter how long we have not been in contact with them that there is an immediate connection with them. They to this day remain more like family than the Riemer's do.

Uncle Dave and Aunt Katherine have both passed on but they will never be forgotten. In my mind's eye I will always be able to see their farmstead and see myself running around the circle that went down a hallway, through the kitchen, then the dining room, into the living room and back to the hall. All the time wondering around which corner Uncle Dave would scare us from next.

Chapter 11

June 18, 2008 — Tubal pregnancy
Adriel: member of God's flock, nurtured of God
Peter: rock, powerful faith

About June 14th, 2008 I started feeling pregnant again. We were excited about this one because the timing was exactly what we had dreamed of as far as the spacing between our first two children. At this time, I was still solely breastfeeding Tirzah but I knew it was still possible that I could have conceived again. I had gone to sleep on the 17th but woke up around 11:30 p.m. with severe pain in my pelvic area.

Rob also woke up when they hit because I cried out in pain and sat up really quickly. At first I thought it was just a muscle spasm but realized very quickly the pain was much more severe than that. I went downstairs to call Health Links, hoping they would assure me it was all okay. I thought moving around would take away the pain. I got downstairs and Rob was basically right behind me fully dressed and carrying Tirzah (just an idea of how long it took me to get downstairs). We skipped the phone call and headed to St. Boniface Hospital.

Rob parked by the doors of Emergency to drop me off. I got out of the car and started towards the doors. Some security staff were outside having a smoke with a patient in a wheelchair. They took one look at me and the patient stood up and the security guard rushed the wheelchair to me and pushed me in with Rob following with Tirzah. The security guard told Rob to move the vehicle when I was admitted and not to worry about it. We spoke with the triage nurse and were immediately brought to a room and the long night began.

I told the doctor I thought I was pregnant. He indicated it was impossible to know this early based on having morning sickness as that would not come till a couple of weeks later. When the blood test came back he came and told us I was indeed pregnant. He seemed surprised, and almost expected us to be. My answer to him was that I knew that. The pain had diminished somewhat by then, so I refused medication just in case it was a viable pregnancy, but in my mind I was sure it wasn't.

Tirzah was as good as gold that night. She slept off and on. Sometime in the early morning she rolled over for the first time. We had to wait for an ultrasound, which was scheduled for about 10:00 a.m. the morning of the 18th. We were hoping for a good report but somehow knew it would not be. While waiting for the ultrasound we did some singing to encourage ourselves. Two of the songs that I remember singing were "Count your blessings" and "Blessed be your name". The ultrasound technician did the ultrasound and then said she would go get the doctor. We knew what that meant. The doctor came in and after a few moments of looking, asked us if this was a planned pregnancy. I think he wondered this because of Tirzah's age and it would probably have been easier for him to tell us that it was an ectopic pregnancy if it was not planned. We told him it was not planned but neither was it unplanned; we wanted this baby.

He then told us it was not to be. The baby was in the fallopian tube. There was already hemorrhaging. I was wheeled back to the emergency room. The doctor came in and explained the options for terminating the pregnancy. Every fiber in my body was screaming no, but I knew that we had no options. The side effects of most of the options carried too much risk for my health and Tirzah's wellbeing. With the chemical method, one of the side effects was possible kidney failure on my part and because of the transference of drugs through the breast milk I would have had to wean Tirzah cold turkey that day. They could also have tried saving the tube but the chance was much greater that another tubal would follow if I ovulated on that side and the next time the situation could possibly be of even greater risk to me. Or they could remove the tube completely. We opted to remove the tube altogether.

With this method I would still be able to nurse Tirzah with no interruption. I did in fact nurse her in pre-op and she was fine until I came out of surgery and I was nursing her again within a half hour of being in my room. I was just warned she might be a little sleepy for a while but that the anesthetic would not harm her.

One other concern was whether she would be allowed to stay with me when I was in the hospital for the next few days.

They said they would accommodate this request but I would need to have someone with me at all times because the nurses could not be responsible for her in any way.

I would have preferred having the baby removed by laparoscopy but because of the internal bleeding they had already discovered with the ultrasound they felt it was best to do it with an incision.

Rob left to make some phone calls and during this time they came to prep me for surgery. I panicked when it appeared that Rob would not be back before they took me to surgery. He did come back in time and the nurse there assured me that if he had any trouble with Tirzah they would help and if she got hungry they would have something to give her. During the surgery my Aunt Evelyn came to stay with Rob, which he appreciated very much. I was not aware that she had come until after the surgery was over.

I went in for surgery about 1:30 p.m. and was back in my room at about 3:00 p.m. I was very thirsty because I had had nothing but a few pieces of ice and a mint or two since the evening before. How good that water tasted. I just had to be careful not to drink too much too fast.

The doctor who performed my surgery did an amazing job of stitching me back up. The scar is so slight that people would not even see it unless they knew it was there. I stayed in the hospital till the 20th, Rob's birthday. Rob spent both nights in the hospital.

During this hospital stay, a chaplain came by to see me. He spoke with me a little and expressed sadness for our loss. He recommended that we name the child. This is the only loss where Rob and I felt very strongly that he had been a boy. With none of the other losses did we have any strong feelings one way or the other.

On the 19th, my Aunt Annie came and on the 20th Rob's Aunt Mary-Anne and Uncle Ed came. They brought me home that afternoon and we celebrated Rob's birthday. Thankfully, Tirzah was as light as she was (5.9 Kg or 13 lbs.) because my doctor told me that I could lift her but nothing heavier for about three weeks. This meant I was able to recover at home without needing someone to care for Tirzah. The physical recovery was much easier than the emotional recovery.

This loss was harder than the first one because as soon as I knew I was pregnant all the memories of the pregnancy with Tirzah, the delivery and the joy of holding a newborn came back to me and I knew this time what I was missing. Oh yeah, and there was the seven months of morning sickness that I almost forgot about. The first time I imagined what it would be like but our imagination is not nearly as strong as the memories of the real thing.

January 21, 2009 — Second miscarriage
Litonya: darting hummingbird, child of God

On January 21st, 2009 I was about three days late with my period and on the day I was going to test I started to bleed. The bleeding started excessively heavy and with severe cramping. After the first few minutes the cramping stopped but the bleeding continued much heavier than what was normal for me. We lost Litonya that day. Another tipoff for me was that Tirzah once again had a yeast infection. She had had one when we lost Adriel as well.

I had a doctor's appointment for Tirzah a few days later and spoke with the doctor about this. She agreed with me that this had been another miscarriage. At this point I was starting to wonder what was wrong with me. It seemed I was losing a larger percentage of pregnancies than would be considered normal. At this time I was still full of hope that we would eventually carry another one to term. The doctor also was starting to wonder if there might be something wrong. But at this time she did not yet make a referral to a specialist.

August 27 – September 16, 2009 — Third miscarriage
Jezaniah: God determines, in God's hands

In August I found myself in Emergency again, knowing I was pregnant. I had done a test that was positive, but a very weak positive. At about five and a half weeks I started spotting heavily. They did the blood work and my hormone level was not matching the number of weeks that I was pregnant. They did an ultrasound and determined it was not a tubal, however I was told I would probably miscarry because the hormone level indicated the pregnancy was in trouble. I went home and about two days later the spotting stopped but the pregnancy symptoms did not.

During the ultrasound we had seen the heartbeat. Something else was mentioned during the ultrasound by the doctor that would later have proved very helpful in treating me more quickly (if I had not had a full term pregnancy). The doctor told me it looked like I had what he called a heart-shaped uterus, like something was attached at the top of it. Because the symptoms of pregnancy did not go away and I had had no clear miscarriage, I was looking forward to the ultrasound in three weeks because I was sure things had straightened themselves out and I was going to carry this one to term. I was starting to show when I went for the follow-up appointment.

Imagine my shock and surprise when the technician told me it was all clear and I was good to go. I asked what she meant and she told me the miscarriage had been complete and I would not need to have a D&C. When I didn't seem to comprehend this, she realized that maybe she needed to call in the doctor. He explained to me I had miscarried Jezaniah sometime between the two ultrasounds. He said he would forward the results from both ultrasounds to my doctor and I should call to make an appointment with her as soon as possible. I was numb. I got to the car and called Rob. He was as shocked as I was.

We were eating supper at about 7:00 p.m. that night when my doctor called me. She could not believe the findings any more than we could. She explained to me that occasionally a mother's body will simply absorb the pregnancy and there will never be an actual miscarriage. When this happens the body continues to believe it is pregnant because the hormones do not go back to pre-pregnancy levels but will continue to be elevated because the trigger to bring them down has not been activated — hence the pregnancy symptoms. She had heard of this but never had she had a patient to whom this had happened. I made an appointment to see her in her office and she decided it was time I went to a fertility specialist because now she was convinced there was a problem that would need further attention if I was to carry to full term again.

I had my first appointment with the fertility specialist in the spring 2010. On the first visit when he took my medical history, I remember telling him what the doctor had said during the first ultrasound about my uterus appearing heart shaped. If only he had taken that statement seriously, I might have had to only have one surgery and it might have happened a lot sooner. Instead, I spent the next couple of months doing a truck load of blood work and had a few more appointments with him.

The blood work showed that there was nothing wrong with my hormones. He then recommended I have a test done where he would inject a dye into the uterus and take some x-rays. The results stumped us both. By this time I did not have a left tube but the liquid was not draining out of my right one either, as if it was entirely blocked. About a week before this test I had lost Nika (my third miscarriage since I had the tubal). If fluid could not enter the right tube at all, how could I have conceived and lost three babies? He almost implied that I might not have actually been pregnant those three times. I left the appointment upset. I was the one that saw the + on the test, not him. At the follow-up appointment he suggested surgery to check for any scar tissue within the tube. We agreed although I was sure that scar tissue was not the problem.

May 24, 2010 — Fourth miscarriage
Nika: belonging to God, purchased

We headed to my parents' for the May long weekend. I knew I was pregnant but the + sign had been very faint and we were sure this was not a good thing. A few weeks before this, we had asked the pastor in the church we were attending at the time if the elders would be willing to anoint us with oil and pray for us. To our amazement and a degree of disbelief, he said he would have to discuss this with the elders and would get back to us. We had no idea that this biblical concept would need to be discussed.

On the Sunday of this long weekend, I approached my old youth leader, who was now one of the two acting pastors in the church that I grew up in, asking if he and some of the elders would pray for us. His response could not have been more different than the pastor in the city. He said they most certainly would. He then said he would quickly round up any elders that were still at church (as this was after the service) and they would meet us at the front of the church. Within five minutes, we were surrounded by four of the elder couples.

We explained why we were asking them to pray and after anointing us with oil, they prayed for us. We knew this in no way ensured I would ever carry another child to term, but I believe this small act gave us the assurance that regardless of what happened we had the support of our Christian brothers and sisters. We had followed what the Bible taught and it was an act of obedience on our part. The irony in all of this is that the church we attended in Winnipeg was a non-denominational church and the one I grew up in was a Mennonite church.

The next day I was feeling extremely tired and very sad. The cramps started and I knew we were losing Nika that morning, which we did. I spent the morning lying in bed and crying. After I lost the baby I went and told Rob. By this time the shock factor was gone. We had been there and done that so many times already that it was more normal to lose a baby than to carry it to term. I think we would have been more shocked if I had actually carried to term. Maybe it was a defence response so we wouldn't feel the pain as deeply.

That afternoon before we headed back to Winnipeg we had a potluck at Aunt Lorna and Uncle Dwight's. We told them we had just lost another one that morning and they were free to tell the pastoral team, as the pastoral team had said they would continue to pray for us and we were free to give them any updates that we wanted to.

Chapter 12

September 2 and 16, 2010 —
Surgery with fertility specialist

I went in for the first surgery on September 2nd, very sceptical because I didn't agree with the doctor's reasoning. After I was out of surgery, he came to see me. He told me he had good news and bad news. First the good news. They had discovered the problem and it was not what they had expected at all. He told me we had a miracle child. I had a condition called a uterine septum. The membrane that split the uterus in two at conception and usually dissolves by birth had not entirely dissolved, leaving me with a loose flap hanging from the top of my uterus. This acted like a natural IUD.

In all his years as a specialist, he had seen this condition quite a number of times but never had the woman carried a full term pregnancy. The bad news was he had not left enough time or had the tools on hand to correct this. He said another surgery would be booked and they would put me on the cancellation list. About four days later I got a call from his office to ask how I was doing. When I said I was doing great, the receptionist told me there had been a cancellation and wondered if I could come in for surgery again on September 16th, exactly two weeks from the first one. I said I could.

Two weeks to the day I went in again and had another surgery to remove the flap. This time my recovery was not as smooth. After surgery I was by and large ignored by the nurses. My blood pressure wasn't stabilizing and even though I had been one of the first ones in for surgery that day, I was the last one to leave and I left at this time only because I told them I was going. The last person had left about two hours before that.

I had been fasting since the night before and by five o'clock I told them I was starting to experience low blood sugar. They finally came over and checked and told me I wasn't but very quickly had juice there for me. I was not impressed with the care. At a little before 7:00 p.m. I asked them if they were planning to keep me overnight. They said no, they were going to release me shortly. I saved them the trouble and said we were leaving now because we needed to pick up Tirzah from the sitter's and I needed to go eat.

There was no reason I should have been kept there that long. If there was a problem with my blood pressure then they should have been actively trying to do something about it, not just letting me lie there an hour on end without checking on me. My recovery at home was much slower than the previous time, but I did have the hope I would now conceive and carry to term within the next year. I went for a follow-up appointment with the specialist about six weeks later and learned how much of a miracle Tirzah actually was.

He said that in his blog communications with the other fertility specialists across Canada and some in the US, not one of them had ever seen a woman with this condition have a full term pregnancy. Tirzah had rewritten the medical books on the condition of uterine septums. He said all the signs that I had had pointed to this condition but because I had a full term pregnancy he had dismissed it. He said that now all the specialists he had communicated with would not dismiss it if in fact there was a full term pregnancy involved.

I remember telling him about what the doctor who had performed last ultrasound had said (about the shape of my uterus and asked if anyone had mentioned that to me or if it had been investigated). When I brought that up again at this appointment he said he remembers me saying it but ignored it because of my full term pregnancy. All that said, I realize now this might all have been discovered a little too late. Looking back I realize I was probably entering pre-menopause at this point and my chances of pregnancy were already greatly reduced.

March 19, 2011 — Fifth miscarriage
Shala: borrowed, dedicated

We informed immediate family and few close friends as soon as I discovered I was pregnant again. The pregnancy test had not been very strong, so we were already anticipating losing another one. We lost Shala on March 19th, 2011, between weeks six to seven . I had not started to really show yet so we were glad about this. At this point we were numb to the fact we had just lost another baby. We felt loss but not enough to really mourn it. Life just continued as normal. It was almost a relief the loss had occurred because that is what we had been expecting. We could no longer face a pregnancy excited about the possibility of a full-term because of the possible disappointment so we took the safer route, believing from the start that God would take this one from us too. And He did.

Chapter 13

Feb 11-12/2012 / May 9/12 — Sixth miscarriage
Rena: peaceful, abiding in God

What a roller coaster. At the beginning of December, I told
Rob that this month was a wash. I had ovulated on the side
where the tubal pregnancy had been. When this happened we
knew my period would come and we didn't have our hopes
up that I might conceive that month. By Christmas morning
I had been not feeling well for about a week. Just so I could
enjoy the Christmas with our families I decided to take a
pregnancy test. I wanted to verify that I was not pregnant. I
did not tell Rob I was taking it. At 5:30 a.m. that morning I
did the test and within a minute there was a very clear plus
sign in the test area before the test was considered finished.

All the previous miscarriages had been a faint positive but
this one was very much there. I burst into tears. As I held
the test, I wept for what felt like a long time as my gaze
was locked in on the plus. In reality it may have been less
than five minutes. When I had finally composed myself (I
thought) I took the test and went to our bedroom where Rob
was enjoying his sleep. He stirred as I entered the room and
as I found his hand and pressed the test into his hand I said

"Merry Christmas" as I burst into tears of joy again. His first response was, "You're kidding." He then told me that when I had told him it was a wash his first thought had been that this is the month God would cause me to conceive.

I started spotting on January 31st, 2012. Fear wanted to get me so bad. During the attacks from the enemy I held on to the fact that God was still God. I listened to the gospel album that we have of the Statler Brothers. The song that really stuck out was the song 'Leaning on the everlasting arms'. The first line of the chorus goes 'Leaning, leaning, safe and secure from all alarm.'

On February 11th I lost Rena after spotting for about two weeks or so we thought. This was such a disappointment. I had already been showing for about four weeks at this point. On February 6th a blood test showed that I was definitely ten and a half weeks pregnant and the doctor stated the spotting was of no concern because of the quantity and the fact that it appeared to be old blood. However, he ordered an ultrasound because of my history of miscarriages. This was just to make sure that everything was all right and see if they could determine the cause of the spotting. He booked an ultrasound for that Thursday, February 9th.

What the ultrasound technician found was not what we were expecting. The doctor was called in. I was informed that the baby measured only six and a half weeks and there was no heartbeat. The doctor asked me if I was sure of my dates and I assured him I was. They did not say it was a miscarriage at this time because they said the size of the baby might have something to do with not finding a heartbeat because of presentation. But because of the differing information between the blood work from four days earlier and the ultrasound more blood work was required. Over the next week and a half I donated blood to the medical profession three times. When it came back the doctor verified that I had a missed miscarriage. A missed miscarriage is when the baby dies but again the trigger in the mothers body is not triggered and the pregnancy 'continues normally'.

On Feb 27th I sent out this email to the Friesen family. I figured this was the easiest way to let them know what was happening without having to make all the calls (the family is large stemming from the fourteen children Grandma Friesen was blessed to have).

"Would you be so kind as to pass this on to the Friesen mailing list? Thanks. (This part was addressed to the faithful uncle who is the middle man to the mass communications for our family.) 'How is everyone doing? I figured that it would be easier to get a mass email sent out to give everyone an update. At the beginning of February I had some spotting that the doctor assured me was not concerning. That said, he sent me for an ultrasound because of my history of miscarriages. When I went for the ultrasound later that week we discovered the baby was four weeks smaller than expected from the blood work and there was no heartbeat found. Further blood work over the next week and a half showed I was losing the baby. About two weekends ago, we believe that we lost the baby. Thank you so much for all your prayers up to this point and for your continued prayers. We do want more children but God has given us peace about what our family status is right now and are confident if there are to be more that God can work that out marvellously in His time (too bad our time doesn't always match His).

Regardless of the circumstances, God is still GOD.'"

At my Wednesday morning Bible study at Church, Kimberley Anhalt approached me and gave me an envelope. She said she had written a poem for me at the end of January and had waited till now to give it to me because it seemed so inappropriate at the time. Now that the pregnancy had taken the turn that it had, she understood what she had penned back then. Once you read it you will understand.

Darlene

Time, it travels and leaves heartaches in its path
With broken wings.
I've walked the roads of simplicity
But sometimes I have to change direction.
For that was not the right way.
Your voice is distant.
In these times, I have to strain to hear you.
Your words fall like rain and I desire to catch them.
This poor girl.
The one you love.
Your daughter
You know my mind and what's inside.
The ocean is deep, with tormented waves
Then silence
The sun glistening off soft ripples in the water.
The aftermath
I can only understand as far as You allow
Trust in concrete and Your Word, the Finisher
I am at a loss without this.
I stay humbled with the blessings.
And grounded with the losses
But still. I pray for more.
Hope is on the horizon!
I see Your face, the eyes of knowledge
And comfort.
So much comfort
I will depend on Your strength.
It is the only way
As February snow falls

It covers the ground
A reminder it is still winter.
Dark days will be here.
A little while longer
My tears, though many have fallen.
Your compassion will dry them
Your love will sustain me

We thought this was the end of the pregnancy until March 1st. My nausea had never totally disappeared but my baby bump did come back on Feb. 11th. On the first of March I told Rob I thought I was getting my period because I was having slight cramps and my stomach was feeling tight. By the time he got home my baby bump was back and the nausea was back. By Friday, I was almost as big as I had been when I had lost our 'last one' a little over two weeks ago.

That night we made a trip to Wal-Mart to get another pregnancy test. We could not wait till Monday when I had a doctor's appointment to follow up on the miscarriage. We got home and I took the test that night and it was positive. Now we didn't know what to think or what to tell people. We contacted a few of our close family and friends, as well as some prayer chains. How thankful we have been for the people that have surrounded us with prayer. On Monday, when I saw my doctor, she was in shock. This was something she had never encountered in her career. She ruled out a lost multiple. This left two options in her mind — either I had gotten pregnant on the rebound or it was a partial miscarriage. She said she had never seen the first option but the signs were not consistent with the second option.

More blood work. This time I was to go four times in a period of two weeks. She said we should see a trend forming to verify which option it might be and then she would send me for an ultrasound after that. As I was leaving she asked me if I couldn't just do things by the book. Looking back I should have told her I was, just not hers. This was the one that God had written for me (us).

Up to this point there had been no real bleeding. The blood work did verify I had indeed lost the baby but the hormone levels were coming down really slowly. My doctor told me it was just a matter of waiting for the hormone levels to drop enough so I would have the actual miscarriage. On March 23rd the bleeding started. I bled fairly heavily for a week, and then I stopped. I thought the miscarriage was now complete. I was wrong. About a week later I bled for a day and did so every two to three days for the next three weeks. This was starting to concern me as it did not seem normal.

On April 2nd, I received a letter from Dad in the mail (written March 25th). Having just finished my miscarriage (or so I thought), the letter could not have come at a more appropriate time. I have included it here:

> My Dearest Darlene & Rob & Tirzah,
>
> You don't know why I am in tears as I am writing this. It is because of a short story I read during lunch in the book — Women at the Well.
>
> This mother during shopping that morning, had just met the third mom and baby set, when she burst into tears. One and a half years earlier she had lost her only child thro' a miscarriage. By now her friends had returned to their "normal" lives.
>
> That morning she was reminded that Moms never get over the loss of a child, even a preborn child.

Of course my thoughts went to you. I could blame myself for not having more acknowledged your multiple "miscarriages", but I would rather think that God in His perfect time had led me to that story and thereby prompted me to write. P.T.L!!

I'm not a mother — and thus do not have a mother's "heart". But it comes to me again, that when we "lost" your brother Daniel Dale, your mommy never really "got over it". I wasn't often reminded of it, because of the way she carried on with life. But there were "telling" moments.

But when Debbie "was so slow" in following you we applied for adoption. We were sure two would be better than one! But when Debbie appeared "on the horizon" we withdrew from further proceedings and cancelled out.

So how is faith in our dear Lord Jesus holding out and carrying you? On your mommy's headstone you and Deb chose the inscription, "Great is Thy Faithfulness." We (I) understand and trust, that His Faithfulness is still there, and still again upholding you! Thank you, Jesus!!

Kathryn Olson — the mother in the above story shares some pointers to help along in coping:

1. Be gentle with yourself.

2. Allow yourself to grieve.

3. Expect emotional up and downs.

4. Embrace the life God has for you.

5. Look for God's comfort (maybe the letter fits in here).

I will close with the prayer she closes her story with:

"Lord, everywhere I go I see pregnant women or children in strollers and yet my arms are still empty. I need your peace, Lord. You have promised to bind up the broken hearted. Give me increased faith to believe that your purpose for me is perfect, even though it is painful. And use what you are teaching me to encourage others. In the name of the Gentle Shepherd, Amen."

Darlene and Rob and Tirzah. Remember "That with God nothing is impossible" P.T.L!! Thanks for showing courage!

Dad

I have not voluntarily held a newborn since about ten months after Tirzah was born. When I have held a child less than six months since then it has been because the mother just put the little one in my arms because they needed to do something. This has happened about three or four times in my memory. I just can't emotionally deal with the feelings of holding a small baby.

On April 22nd, I started bleeding heavier than I had a month ago. On Monday, I called my doctor but it was her day off, so I went to a walk-in clinic. The doctor there called for more blood work and put in a request for an emergency ultrasound. I got the ultrasound on Wednesday, and the technician told me if I had not heard from a doctor by the following Monday I should follow up. The next day I got a call from the walk-in doctor's office and they wanted to see me that morning. I was hit with a wave of fear. I think this was a normal response of anyone who is waiting for test results. She was hoping to get me a D&C within the next day or two. She made a gynaecologist appointment for Monday. By my appointment at the gynaecologist on April 30th I had stopped bleeding again. She told me she was going to get a D&C for me as soon as possible.

She also asked me if we were done trying because if we were, she could do a hysterectomy. This was not an option at this point. As hopeless as we felt right then, we knew we wanted to have another child. She got me an emergency appointment for the next day and we managed to arrange for childcare on short notice. When I got home later that day there was a message on our machine saying the appointment was cancelled and they had booked me for a May 9th appointment. This was extremely disappointing. Another week and a half of spotting and nausea followed.

Sometime between finding out that we had lost Rena and the D&C I had trouble sleeping one night. I started talking to God and asking for a sign that He still cared. He gave me a vision that night. The picture He gave me was of our whole family. Rob, myself and our eight children were standing together in heaven praising God. Our family was standing around us and I was holding Rena who was the size of a baby. The children were all different sizes from Kipp who was taller than Tirzah to Rena who was in my arms. I fell asleep comforted that night.

On May 9th, my in-laws came in to take me to the hospital and to look after Tirzah. Rob was out of town for the night with his job and so they had agreed to stay the night as well. I got to the hospital and was booked into pre-op. After they had given me a bed, the nurse looking over my chart asked me if they could call a chaplain to talk to me. I was a little puzzled when she told me this was their practice.

Mark came to my bed and expressed his condolences on our loss and then I understood. They were treating this as a death and rightfully so. This was just a little unusual in my way of thinking because of the general mindset the culture has toward the unborn. He gave me a package they have put together for grieving parents and talked with me for a while.

As we talked, the grief I was burying just came gushing out. He asked me if the baby had a name and I told him her name was Rena, named by Tirzah. Since October, Tirzah had an imaginary friend she referred to as Rena. For all our investigating we could not find a person in her life that had that name or even a similar name. The last time she ever referred to Rena was when I told her one night that Jesus had taken our baby to heaven and the baby was dead.

Her response went something like this — "Oh, why?" When I told her I didn't know she said, "Will Jesus give us another one then?" We never heard about Rena again. He asked me what we wanted to have done with Rena's remains. I told him I had not expected that question and had not discussed this with my husband but I was pretty sure he would agree with me in the decision to release them to the hospital as we had with the tubal. He then encouraged me with scripture and prayed with me before he left.

I was rolled into surgery a few minutes later and came to about forty-five minutes later. Within the hour, Dad and Mom Wiebe together with Tirzah came to pick me up. After surgery my bleeding stopped immediately and all pregnancy symptoms disappeared. The fog in my head lifted and my energy came back. Where before it was all I could do to look after the two children I babysat, the first day I had them the next week I made bread, mowed two lawns, and still wasn't as exhausted as before.

A miracle took place that day. About an hour after I got home I realized I was missing my rings. I was sure they had somehow fallen out of my purse into the bottom of the bag that I had my stuff in. I called the hospital in a panic. I got the desk of the day-op station and the lady on the phone told me a custodian had happened to see my ring in the bag before he had thrown it out. When I told her that there had been two bands. I heard her immediately called the custodian to tell him there had been two rings.

She then told me he was going to see if they could find it as they knew which bags had come from the area. She was not too hopeful though. A little later she called me back and said the same custodian had found the engagement ring as well. We had supper and I went to pick it up. I was able to meet the man and thank him personally for his service that went above and beyond what was expected of him (for being attentive on the job) and gave him a few chocolates. He had a tear in the corner of his eye and I turned to go. God gave me a sign that He still cared about me and the things in my life, small or big. I am not sure if the miracle of the rings was a big or small thing.

During the last part of April and the month of May our church was split into small groups. We were all doing the forty days of community Bible studies by Rick Warren. When they started I felt like I was a fraud. I had nothing left to give anyone; I was strictly in survival mode and resented anyone who wanted anything from me (except Tirzah). I felt I did not have a clear head and any decision that had to be made was a huge ordeal to me.

Sometimes I was in pj's half the day because I didn't know what to wear. Many mornings I would go back to bed after Rob left for work. By the end of each day I was exhausted and just wanted to cry. At this point I was ready to pack up all the baby stuff and give it away. This was the first time I had felt so hopeless about having more children. The third week we were talking about belonging together and how love always protects, trusts, hope and perseveres. I thought I was that kind of person for those around me but it hit me that I also needed to allow those around me to be that for me.

I knew I was a mess inside and yet I was pretty sure not many others knew it, aside from my friend Judy. I could accept others as equally valuable and important despite their ' valley moments' but somehow I could not see myself as valuable or important to a group if I could not contribute in any way. Over the next couple of weeks I built up the courage to tell our small group I needed them and I could at this point offer nothing in return. They reached out to me and I experienced for one of the first times how it felt to be at the receiving end without needing to give anything in return from people other than family. They set up a prayer chain for me and Rob so there was at least one couple praying for us every day over the next two weeks.

On August 26th Pastor Keith had a few prophesies he verbalized on Sunday morning. There was one that struck both me and Rob, because it was describing us. "And there is also a lady here that would like to have a bulge. You would like to be pregnant. Now you are married, it is not an unmarried situation: you are married and God is speaking to you about fruitfulness. A barrenness that has been upon you for five years you've been waiting and He says, 'I'm the God who is going to cause fruitfulness to come to you' and by next year you'll say — beginning of September — that God was faithful to me. Okay?"

I have been hopeful so many times that I have developed a skepticism about this area of my life so I will not be hurt so badly. I knew this could be describing us, but I thought it could possibly be someone else he was speaking to. After all, what made me think that we were the only ones struggling in this area and after all I had been pregnant in those five years. Rob told me to not analyze it so much because he firmly believed that it was for us.

October 17th, I had my Uncle Abe (my Dad's brother) and Aunt Olga down for lunch before they headed back to B.C. As they were leaving Uncle Abe asked me out of the blue if we still wanted more children. I said yes and he asked me if he could pray for us. Now understand that many people have prayed for us and so far nothing has happened. I said yes and in my heart I am thinking it cannot hurt but it won't help either.

After he finished praying, he paused for a bit and then said, "By this time next year you will have another baby." I was shocked and Pastor Keith's words came back to mind. Uncle Abe had no way of knowing what had been said that Sunday morning. Rob had told a few people about the prophesy but I chose not to. I determined that if the words came true for us I would share them then as a testament to God being faithful to what He said He would do.

Aunt Olga added after he had finished praying, "You know he has only said those words to one other couple, and they went on to have one within that year and another eight followed." Even with these two separate prophesies I was still in self-defence mode. I started wondering if my unbelief would make it not happen if it was actually meant to happen. God brought to mind the story of Sara. She laughed and I am sure it was in unbelief. A year later she was holding her biological son. God said to me, "If these words were from me, there is nothing you can do to prevent me from causing them to happen. I do not need your belief to accomplish what I have said I will do."

So I continued in my unbelief and knew God was not at all bothered by it. On November 29th, Tirzah woke up cheerful as usual. First she greeted me with her imitation of the baby Jaguar from Diego. After a little snuggle, she told me her baby sister was in Mommy's tummy. I was a little taken aback. She had in the past asked for a baby but never had she directly told me something like this. When I asked her what she meant, she explained. There was a baby in my tummy and after it was done growing it would come out.

Where she got this info I have no idea, but to her it seemed so matter of fact. I just wasn't sure what to make of this in light of the other two prophesies. I was gathering that she had a very vivid dream that night and wonder if it was one given her from God. It came at an interesting time because I knew I was not at this point pregnant but if the first words of prophesy were true then I would have to get pregnant this month or next.

How often I have wished God would speak to me in ways like this but when it happens it is funny how my natural inclination is to dismiss it. As I think about this, I can't help thinking about people in Bible times who had Jesus right there and they didn't believe. It shows that people who say they will believe when they see miracles or hear from God, may never see these because God knows who will believe. It seems to me when God shows Himself in this way it is most often to those who have never even put out this 'fleece'. I think this is because those will see the miracle in it and give God the glory.

Chapter 14

It was now April 5th, 2013. The time has come and gone for the three prophesies. I was still not pregnant. I could accept that the prophesy at church was not about us. It is the other two I have had a very hard time accepting. Those were given specifically to me, so what is up with that? I believed that uncle Abe is not one to say things like that without really believing it came from God. And why would God put the idea in Tirzah's head? This spring was hard emotionally because of this. In February, I thought I was pregnant because I continued to have many of the symptoms (nausea, tender breasts, sore mouth, smelly urine, tiredness, weird dreams, etc.) that come with being pregnant after I had my period.

By now my periods were only lasting about twenty-four to thirty-six hours. When a pregnancy test was negative I was confused and then I started getting really bloated like I was pregnant. I called my doctor's office and asked to get a blood pregnancy test. That came back negative too. I then made an emergency appointment with my doctor because I thought I was losing it. When I saw her she talked with me and explained I was having symptoms of peri-menopause. Our chances of having another one were slim to none the way my hormones were. She recommended hormone replacement therapy.

I told her I would prefer a hysterectomy. I just wanted this to end. I believe the pills would just address the symptoms and not the problem. I didn't want the emotional ups and downs anymore. That way I wouldn't have my period anymore and the symptoms I was experiencing all the time would be gone. It was like a constant reminder I was not pregnant but taunting me with the symptoms. I went home and went straight to the Internet to find out if there was a natural remedy to this major hormonal imbalance.

I started taking some herbs right away because I had them in the house. After about two and a half months they have become my lifeline to sanity. Why is God not listening to us? In March, some dear friends of ours who have had similar challenges as us in the area of children lost another child after ten weeks of bed rest and numerous other challenges. At about twenty-two weeks gestation, little Skyler lived for forty minutes before the Lord took him home. When I heard this I cried for them and for us. I had a great big pity party. When I saw Jen the next day we had a good cry together. I just remember saying to her it was not fair.

I might as well be honest about the situation. I am sure she felt the same way and I was not so spiritual that I am going to try to smooth things over and give some pat answers. Them losing another baby just really sucked and it reminded me of all the ones we had lost. In March, Rob and I agreed to make one last ditch attempt. On day twelve of my cycle I started fasting by not eating anything except at the times I was taking the herbs. I knew I needed those herbs and taking them without eating would have made me sick. I fasted for three days.

I called my friend Judy and told her what we were doing and asked her to pray with us. During this time we also took a double dose of vitamin E about an hour before we had sex and we had sex every two days until day eighteen. On day fourteen we put in a video in for Tirzah and went to our bedroom. After we had had sex, we were snuggling a bit and we just started praying sentence prayers. When we were done, I just felt like we had our answer and that God had heard. During that time of fasting I had been pleading with God that He give us another child. Now I just had to wait to see what the answer was.

I got my period on March 31st, 2013. His answer was "No", and it was just like I was able to accept that Tirzah was going to be an only child. Since then others have told us not to give up hope. I have just told them that if they feel like we should have hope, then they can hope for us because we cannot hope anymore. We would accept with open arms another child if God would bless us with one but we were no longer trying to conceive and in May we planned to tackle the difficult job of cleaning all the baby stuff out of the basement. For our own sanity we cannot keep living in the possibility. There has to be a closing point in all this.

May 8, 2013 — Seventh miscarriage
Mara: bitter

I miscarried our ninth child (eighth loss) May 8th. This came as no surprise. When the test showed positive on the morning of April 27th I was shocked and upset. Rob and I had talked about what our next step was and we were leaning toward a hysterectomy. We were also making plans to empty our basement within the next month. The next few days were hard because we spent the whole time wondering when we would lose this one. Neither of us talked as if I was going to have a full term baby, we were both very emotionally detached.

Our prayer was always that we would have the strength to go through another loss. I hoped it would happen sooner rather than later, as I was again experiencing morning sickness and had a history of showing really early. We told a few close friends and some family, knowing we needed the prayer support. After we lost Mara, we again discussed whether we would do something permanent or if we were just going to continue on in this pattern of conceiving and losing. Every pregnancy is a child and my heart has lost eight now.

What is God expecting me to do? I know in my head that I can trust Him, but I am human too and my heart is numb with grief (to the point where a miscarriage is a relief). Emotionally this was taking a toll on me in ways that not many people understood. It was also taking a toll on my body. Up to April 2012, I was always told my teeth were solid and in very good condition. In October 2012, I had eight cavities. In half a year I developed eight fairly large cavities and even though the dentist says it is not my successive pregnancies and losses, I am not convinced. I have up to that point had seven fillings, five having been there since I was fifteen years old. I have not changed my brushing habits and there have not been any major changes in diet.

On May 10th we brought my cat to my parents' farm because she had some ongoing health challenges that were starting to cost us more than we could afford. I had had her for seven and a half years. I shed more tears over losing her than the miscarriage. Even though sometimes it seemed like the cat was only a make work project, now that she was gone I realize how much she meant to me. Many times she was a warm body that was content to be petted and I now realize how therapeutic this was for me in times of discouragement and loss. Why did she have to start throwing up in this past half year? There have already been days when I want to bring her back, even if I have to clean up after her all day.

I feel like Naomi did returning to Bethlehem, empty handed with Ruth by her side. Ruth 1: 20-21 says, "But she said to them, 'Do not call me Naomi; call me Mara, for the Almighty has dealt very bitterly with me. I went out full, and the LORD has brought me home again empty. Why do you call me Naomi, since the LORD has testified against me, and the Almighty has afflicted me?'" I have named this baby Mara, because like Naomi I feel that the God has dealt bitterly with me. My brain is in a fog (trying to protect itself I think), so as I tried to decide how to deal with my life I was sure of one thing: regardless of what we decided to do, hysterectomy or leave it, I was not in agreement with our decision. It seemed like there was no win-win here, either decision was a lose-lose in our minds.

I went to see the obstetrician/gynaecologist by myself. Rob could not make it. This was hard but life happens. We probably wouldn't have made the decision right then anyway. Dr. Seager was very good. She explained to me what some of the options were and the best ones in her mind were getting my tubes clipped (a day surgery) or Rob going in for a vasectomy (a day surgery) rather than a hysterectomy (a six week recovery). I left the office information in hand. After much discussion and prayer, we decided to call and make an appointment for a tubal ligation. We just needed to wait until I have cycled again so we are sure that there isn't a pregnancy. Once the appointment is made we will need to start using protection to make sure I stay that way — not pregnant.

On July 23rd I finally went to see an infant loss counsellor. This was hard for me to do because I had worked with this organization before and it was in a way humbling to walk through their doors as a client. I had helped others deal with unwanted pregnancies and now I was simply overwhelmed with unwanted miscarriages. I was nervous and unsure about the appointment. It went well though and I felt loved and cared for by someone whom I had worked with almost a decade ago on the crisis line. I will probably go back.

One thing she said to me stood out in my mind. After I had talked for a bit, she told me I was dealing with two griefs right now. The grief of so many losses and the grief of choosing to close the door to more pregnancies. She said that in my heart I still wanted more children but the losses were so heavy that my heart was broken. Each of these griefs on their own was large but the two together would tear anyone apart. She didn't try to talk me out of the decision we have made to have my tubes clipped.

On August 4th I went into Emergency again because I was having all the pregnancy symptoms again and this time there was a great deal of pain in my pelvic area on the right side (the side that still had the fallopian tube). Blood tests confirmed I was definitely not pregnant, so I was booked for an ultrasound for the Tuesday the 6th. They were checking for ovarian cysts. The ultrasound revealed that my ovaries were fine but they checked for kidney stones because I was already there. I concluded the things my body was experiencing were related to peri-menopause and the psychological fear that I would have another tubal (although at this point I would have seen it as somewhat of a blessing because that would mean I would have surgery to remove the tube and then I would know for sure that God was saying we had what He had planned). On Saturday when we had been out at my parents' place I had asked Mom to pray for us because that was the day I had the most pain. She told me maybe it was time to do something about this emotional rollercoaster. I told her we had decided just this last week that I was going to get an appointment for a tubal ligation.

Looking back now I realize that because of my hormonal state of mind I need to be much more aware of the stresses in my life and increase the dose of herbs I'm taking accordingly.

I think I should have been taking more herbs during the time my cousin was living with us. She stayed with us for about five weeks. She works in Africa as an ESL teacher and needed a place to stay till her wedding, which took place in Canada. I got more involved in the wedding planning than I had anticipated, due in part to the fact that I felt I needed to because otherwise it would have landed on an aunt's plate, who was already doing much more than I was.

I was coming off a low time because of having stopped taking the herbs while pregnant in April/May. I had just gotten to the point where I was feeling quite good and then I got pregnant and stopped taking the herbs because I wasn't sure if it was okay to take them while pregnant. As soon as I miscarried Mara, I started taking the herbs again but the damage was done. It took a while before they got the hormones balanced again. My cousin showed up just as they were starting to balance somewhat, and the extra stress did me in again because I was still trying to figure out how to balance the stress factor and the amount of herbs needed.

I had a doctor's appointment on September 16th to book the tubal ligation. The paper work was filled out and the pre-op blood tests were ordered. She said she still had some openings the next week. I was excited about this because of the timing with my cycle. I was expecting my period by the end of the week and then I would not have a chance to get pregnant before the next Wednesday. My one fear was that I was already pregnant, even though I did not have the normal symptoms.

I requested she also order the blood work for a pregnancy test, just to be on the safe side because I have a history of getting pregnant exactly when the doctors tell me I can't or when we are trying not to get pregnant. Since the appointment earlier in the week I started having symptoms of pregnancy. I was sure these were again either attached to peri-menopause or brought on psychologically. I guess I at this point had a view of God that was a little skewed. I thought that it would be just like God to make it work this time, when I was at the point of really not wanting another pregnancy (baby).

Tirzah was already getting to the age where we were able to do a lot of things that a baby would interfere with. And at this time I felt I didn't want to deal with all the baby things again. In the fall session at Woman of Worth (a group of ladies that meet every Wednesday morning at our church) I had started a study by Beth Moore called Believing God. The premise was that many of us believe in God but do we really believe Him. It was the only study out of the six they offered that I felt really pulled to. I decided not to do the homework for a number of reasons. One is that I always did the homework in the past for the Beth Moore studies but never really got a lot out of it. I didn't follow her train of thought and felt that the homework lessons had no real connection to the DVD session.

The second reason this time and the bigger one was that I know I'm on a journey of healing from the grief and pain I have been through these last six years. I did not want to make myself busy with homework that would take away from what God wanted to do in the area of my life that needed healing right now. I was going to continue journaling on my own and see where God would lead me.

My surgery date was originally booked for September 25th. A few days later the receptionist called me and told me that some of the time the doctor had been slotted at the Victoria Hospital had been taken away and my appointment was one of the ones bumped to October 23rd. I was in tears. This was not what I wanted to hear. I knew at this point I was not pregnant and everything had come together so nicely I thought it was almost too good to be true. Apparently it was.

The next month was a hard month. I was scared this would be the month I would get pregnant again and the surgery would be cancelled. I was scared I would then lose it again just before the surgery date and be struck waiting another month or two for a surgery spot. True to form I started having pregnancy symptoms again and felt quite sick for about two weeks. I requested blood work be done again just to make sure I wasn't pregnant and these symptoms were again just hormonal and psychological. I was relieved when I got the results the next day that surgery was on. It was bittersweet in the sense that deep down inside I would love to have another child, but more than wanting another child I did not want another loss.

Now would come the task of starting the cleaning out process and getting rid of the baby stuff occupying about two-thirds of our storage area. This would bring its own challenges, but first things first — get the surgery over with.

On October 20th, we were on our way home from visiting Rob's parents when we started talking about cats. I'm not sure how the conversation got started but I think the root of it was that we had visited friends who had a seven month old kitten. We had watched Tirzah play with the kitten; they had had a lot of fun. The friends asked us if we would consider taking their kitten because they were thinking of getting rid of it. On the trip home, Rob was finally able to talk me into the possibility of a kitten for Tirzah. If we couldn't give her a sibling, at least we could get her a cat. After seeing her with the kitten on the weekend I knew she would love to have a kitten to play with.

We gave the friends a call and said we would consider taking Garfield. After thinking and talking it through however, we thought maybe getting a younger kitten would be better because then Tirzah and it might bond better and it would be easier to train it the way we wanted to. Garfield also had a bad habit of biting and I was scared that this might be a problem when Tirzah tried to play more hands-on with him.

That evening we got home and I went onto Kijiji to see what was available there. We found two possibilities but both had been taken already. After Rob went to bed I looked one more time and saw a kitten I just had to have. I responded to the ad right away and hoped I was the first one because the ad was only three minutes old. The kitten was free but the owner was asking ten dollars for delivery. He responded by the next morning and said the kitten was ours. We were not sure when it was best to tell Tirzah about the kitten, because we were unsure when he would be coming by on Tuesday.

We told her Monday night so that Rob could see her reaction. We showed her the picture on Kijiji and asked her if she liked the kitten. She looked at it and promptly asked if we were getting that kitten. When we said yes she hugged us and thanked us so much for getting her a kitten. She of course wanted to get it right then, but we told her it would come tomorrow. He delivered the kitten on the 22nd around supper time. We let Tirzah decide what to name him from the two names we had chosen — Duke or Radar. She chose Duke.

He settled right in and by the end of the evening looked like he had been at our place all his life. The first night he came upstairs with us on his own and slept on Tirzah's bed. The next morning he came downstairs with Rob and myself. Shortly after Rob left he started crying (a first). He disappeared shortly after that and a little later Tirzah was coming downstairs calling Duke to follow her. I asked her why she was up so early and she said Duke had woken her up. After she was down he stopped his crying. The two became friends quickly. I'm glad we got another cat. I have already found that its good therapy for me too.

I had the surgery on October 23rd. It was a hard day. It was a conflicting day for my feelings. I regretted making the decision to end our family and the next moment I was relieved there would not be another loss. From here on in, when I have pregnancy symptoms I will know they are just menopause related. Rob's parents came to our house to look after Tirzah and the two children I babysit. Things went well there even though the two children had never seen them before. I was glad about that.

My recovery did not go as well as it had in the past. I was much more dizzy and nauseous than previously and had a very sore throat. My blood pressure was fine though, so that was a bonus. When they first took it after surgery they thought it was a little low, but I told them it was about what it was normally. (Before I had gone in for surgery it had been a bit higher than normal, but even then they had thought it was on the low side.) They finally let me leave the hospital about an hour later than they had originally told me before surgery. When I got home I lay on the couch most of the evening, trying not to move. When I did, I got very nauseous and regretted moving.

Rob took Tirzah to Ballet class by himself. They were a little late but Tirzah had really enjoyed herself anyway. Debbie came over to be with me while they were away. I called Lorna and cried to her a little. She suggested I take some Gravol. Rob found some children's Gravol in our medicine cabinet and after taking double the dose recommended for a twelve year old, I started feeling better. I slept well that night. I was supposed to have someone with me for twenty-four hours after surgery but I was on my own the next morning when Rob left for work.

I got the house tidied at least, but it took much longer than it usually would. My abdomen felt very sore and bruised. I was also having a lot of gas pains because of the air they put in as part of the surgery. But "this too shall pass". Our weekend company arrived at 3:00 that afternoon. Sam and

Judy, friends from Bible School and my support over the last few years, arrived from Surrey to spend a couple of days in Winnipeg. They were here to visit us and a couple who were working for the same mission organization they are with. I have looked forward to this visit so much. The timing may have seemed off, but I think it was a godsend.

Their presence alone gives me encouragement. When you have been with them you are refreshed because they are not takers but givers in our relationship. Even though this is only the second time I've seen them since Bible School, it seems our friendship has been able to thrive on phone calls.

Now came the job of sorting through the baby stuff and seeing what we would keep and what we would sell, and if we were selling, how much we would sell it for. So far this was going much easier than I thought. As I went through stuff it has been so factual. It's like I lost all the feelings attached to the things. The evening after I sorted through the maternity clothes though I did some crying. I guess the thought of never feeling a baby inside of me was hard to deal with. I remembered how when I was pregnant I felt somewhat empowered and the warm fuzzies I got when I saw the ultrasound pictures and felt Tirzah's movements.

Even though I had been so morning sick, I enjoyed the other aspects of pregnancy more and those are the ones I seemed to remember. The last two sessions with Beth Moore's "Believing God" referred to the passage in scripture about us speaking to the mountain and it being removed. Her interpretation of this passage was refreshing. She says sometimes God will remove the mountain but sometimes He won't. When He does not it is not necessarily because we do not have enough faith. When it is not removed we need to just start climbing, because when we get to the top we will see the glory of God like we could not have if He had just removed it for us.

It could be that God wanted to reveal Himself to us in a greater way and it was part of the growth that He wanted for us. Another option she shared the second week is that He might split the mountain so we can walk through. The problem is still there but He makes a way through the midst of it and gives us the strength for the journey. As the weeks go on, I am convinced this was the study for me and just these two sessions alone without the homework are what I needed to be encouraged in my walk up and over or through my mountain that God has chosen not to remove.

Right then, I was at a place where the challenges in my life were great enough without being challenged in a Bible study. I needed the cheerleading part to keep on fighting the good fight to get past the present struggle. I felt like Rob and I were coming to a new place in our lives as we accepted our one child family as our new reality and we stopped living in our dreams (and disappointments) of a large family. We were starting to move forward with joy (eventually) instead of looking backwards and being sad about the children we had lost. I was not even thinking about God being able to add to our family if He would choose to by a miracle, but believed this was the final number and this was the number God has for us.

Chapter 15

On December 7th my cousins came by and picked up some of the baby stuff that they wanted. This was hard. Seeing the first of the baby stuff leave our house was extremely emotional. I cried only once when they were here, which surprised me because I thought it might be a lot more. I know they will use these things and make many memories with them as well. They have waited nine years for this child. They had the exact opposite problem than we did, not able to conceive. Now that some of the stuff has left that I would deem necessary if we had another baby, I am ready to see the rest of the stuff sell. I think the initial stuff leaving was probably the most emotional because of the shock and it is always harder to take that first step in an action that is so emotionally charged.

What will the final chapter look like for me? I am not yet sure. Looking back I can tell you that the story does not look like anything I would have written back when I was eighteen. I would have left out the parts about the difficulties I had in my working career, getting married so late in life, and having lost my eight babies. Something I wouldn't even have dreamed of putting in was writing a book. After all, I just about failed English in high school.

I do know a few things that will be in the rest of the journey. There will still be hardships. I am promised that as a follower of Christ. I will always remember the eight precious babies I never held, but I will by the grace of God not keep looking back at the loss but rather move forward.

We have plans to paint our daughter's room purple (she chose that colour) because we are now seeing it as her room and her personal space. A space she will never share with another, so it is time to make it reflect the owner. It is a small step but every great journey starts with a step.

In October we had some family photos taken by my brother. This Christmas we will be sending out Christmas cards for the first time. This is another big step forward because we had wanted to do this a few times already and we never did because we were either just pregnant again, or were getting over the loss of a baby and couldn't get ourselves to send out anything.

There will still be many days that I will be sad, but as time passes I know that they will become fewer and my life will move on as I accept more fully the reality that God gave us one daughter. I will spend more time in doing what I can to help her reach her full potential.

I will choose to allow myself to become vulnerable, so that I might be able to give another women hope that they too can keep moving when their world has just fallen apart with the loss of a child or yet another child.

Willie Robertson said at the end of one of the episodes of Duck Dynasty, "We tend to attach memories to things and then hang onto those things. And sometimes those things are the very things that keep us from making new memories." I have found that regardless of whether or not we keep the things, the memories don't go away and letting go of some of those things that we hang onto so tight may be hard at first but once you start the process gets easier. And as stuff goes, I have discovered a new freedom to move on.

My hope with this book is that it will be an encouragement to others; not just those who have lost children both born and unborn, but also those who know these people. Grief is a very confusing thing because it comes with so many faces. This makes it hard for those who are in the centre of it to clearly understand what they need or are wanting because these things change moment by moment and are so different from person to person.

If two people living in the same house are experiencing the same grief it is even more complicated because of this. That is in my opinion why grief can cause a divorce to take place. That is why in my journey, I never went to my husband as my main support during these long years. I knew he was also grieving but his grief looked so different than mine. He would possibly have cracked under the pressure of dealing with his own grief and being my main support during these years because I know that during this time I was a very needy person.

It wasn't that we never talked or cried together as we faced yet another loss. We shared and held each other many times during our losses but I did not require of him at any time to fully carry me as well. At times when I needed to talk the heavy stuff I called my two friends and went to God with it. I know that many times in my journey grief has looked like anger and I am not sure I or those around me understood this. Now that I know this it is reassuring to know that when I feel this emotion rising what it actually is and am more able to correctly categorize it.

One thing that I have done in this process of life and continue to do is pick my confidante friends carefully. When picking the friends, I have chosen those that I felt were able to stand with me. I was looking for women who would be supportive and pray for me but who I was sure would be able to not take the problems on personally. They also needed to be in a strong place in their lives, so the weight of my situation would not be the last straw on a camel's back.

I have two friends who probably know so much about me right now that I will need to keep them close for life. By not necessarily randomly telling everyone who asked about it a lot of information, I never had a need to keep a large number of people informed all the time. Then I was not having to retell things that hurt on the inside continually. This may have hurt a few people on the way if they perceived themselves to be the only one out of the loop and I am sorry for that, but I needed to keep myself in a safe place so I could eventually find healing. For those who know someone that is grieving I hope that if they did not understand the heart of the bereaved that they understand it a little better now. The ones in grief are not always looking for answers or solutions that you may feel you are expected to give.

The problem is that silence has become something very uncomfortable in our society. Most often the grieving just need a shoulder to cry on, the ability to talk without any feedback, a pat on the back to let them know you care, or simply sitting with them in silence for a while. After my tubal pregnancy the church I was attending at the time delivered us three suppers, and my sister volunteered to come clean my house for me once. Those acts of service towards us made us feel so loved and cared for. Even though you are not saying a word, often your simple acts of caring and listening speak louder than anything you could verbally say. The problem with grief is that it is not problem that can be fixed. With time it will mostly heal, but it will never entirely go away. No amount of words will make a difference.

To those that are grieving right now, I just want to say: be gentle with yourself and know that time has a way of changing perspective. Find a friend (or two) that is able to be your strength for a while, and most of all turn to God. Sing songs about God's goodness especially when you don't feel like it. God doesn't change even when we go through hard times. Regardless of what happens in our lives God is still God. When we choose to praise God even in the hard times, it is amazing how the feelings eventually follow your words. It will not make the sad things go away but it will make them easier to bear.

One child that we have been blessed to hold and eight children that we will never hold in our arms but will hold forever in our hearts

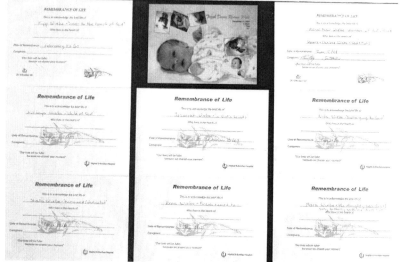

This is a poster that I made with the 'certificates of remembrance' I received from the St. Boniface Hospital in Winnipeg. I filled one out for every child and created this poster. I also included a birth announcement sent out when Tirzah was born. The poster was another step in my grieving/healing process.

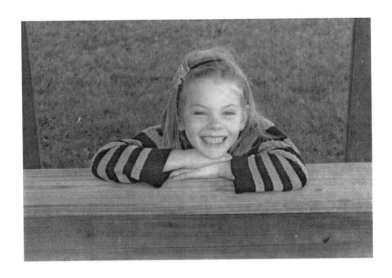

This is our miracle daughter at almost six years old. She has lived up to her name and been a pleasant child who is loved by all. She has a ready smile for anyone and will be quick to announce to me that she has a new friend at the playground — a child who was alone and needed a friend and someone she has never seen before. Her love for life is infectious and the need to keep up with her energy will keeping me young for many years to come.

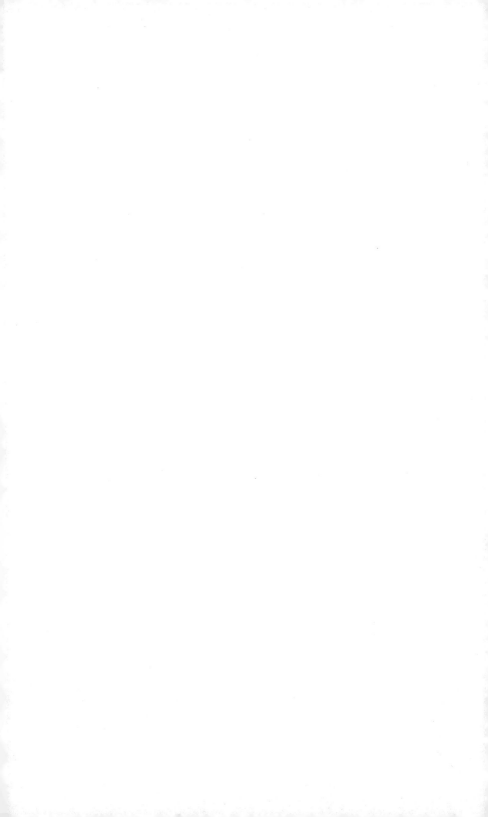

CPSIA information can be obtained at www.ICGtesting.com
Printed in the USA
LVOW06s0220230814

400492LV00002B/15/P